KU-267-865

ADVANCE PRAISE FOR

THE LOW-FODMAP DIET COOKBOOK

'The recognition that FODMAPs are responsible for symptoms in many people with IBS was a major breakthrough in the management of IBS. IBS has been a daunting problem for patients and their physicians for years. We have seen many drugs and different dietary fads come and go. This solution for many patients with IBS is based on sound scientific and physiological mechanisms. Combined with good medical care that includes testing for coeliac disease, small intestinal bacterial overgrowth, and fructose and lactose intolerance, the low-FODMAP diet can be individualized, liberalized, and tailored to each patient. In this book, Sue Shepherd provides a great deal of information on how to make the low-FODMAP diet a delight.'

– PETER H. R. GREEN, MD, Professor of Clinical Medicine and Director
of the Celiac Disease Center at Columbia University

'*The Low-FODMAP Diet Cookbook* is a kitchen essential for anyone following the low-FODMAP diet. Sue Shepherd's easy writing style will make you feel like you have your best friend in the kitchen cooking alongside you. However, this particular best friend has in-depth knowledge about how certain foods will affect your digestive system, as Sue Shepherd has been the driving force behind the diet. The recipes included are lush and decadent, showing you that the low-FODMAP diet need not be one of deprivation. You will see that you can enjoy delicious meals without worry that they will cause you unwanted digestive distress.'

– DR. BARBARA BOLEN, IBS Expert for About.com and coauthor
of *The Everything® Guide to the Low-FODMAP Diet*

SELECTED PRAISE FOR

THE COMPLETE LOW-FODMAP DIET

'This detailed, yet easy-to-understand book [on] a scientifically proven dietary treatment that's rapidly gaining recognition around the world . . . is the roadmap for eliminating problem foods and reintroducing items to find the customized food plan that works specifically for you. More than 80 gut-friendly, gluten-free recipes are included.'

– *LIVING WITHOUT*

'The low-FODMAP diet has revolutionized my practice and has helped so many of my patients. If you suffer from irritable bowel syndrome and choosing food is a challenge, this splendid book is a must-have survival guide. Begin your journey back to good gut health by using food as medicine.'

– GERARD E. MULLIN, MD, Associate Professor of Medicine
and Director of Integrative GI Nutrition Services at
The Johns Hopkins University School of Medicine, and coauthor of
The Inside Tract: Your Good Gut Guide to Great Digestive Health, http://thefoodmd.com

'For those with coeliac disease who continue to have digestive issues, *The Complete Low-FODMAP Diet* is a must-read. [It does] a tremendous job both in identifying the foods responsible for digestive distress and in offering a personalized approach to a balanced diet free from those triggers. With science-based information and easy-to-follow recipes, this book delivers the *why* and *how* that people are looking to know.'

– ALICE BAST, President of the National Foundation for Celiac Awareness (NFCA)

'A complete reference guide about the low-FODMAP diet. The book offers evidence that supports the use of the low-FODMAP diet to manage digestive symptoms, especially IBS. The authors walk you through precise diets, recipes, and menus to put the diet into practice. The recipes are easy to follow and the illustrations are quite breathtaking. I strongly recommend this book for all IBS sufferers.'

– JEFFREY D. ROBERTS, MS Ed, BSc, Founder of IBS Self Help and Support Group

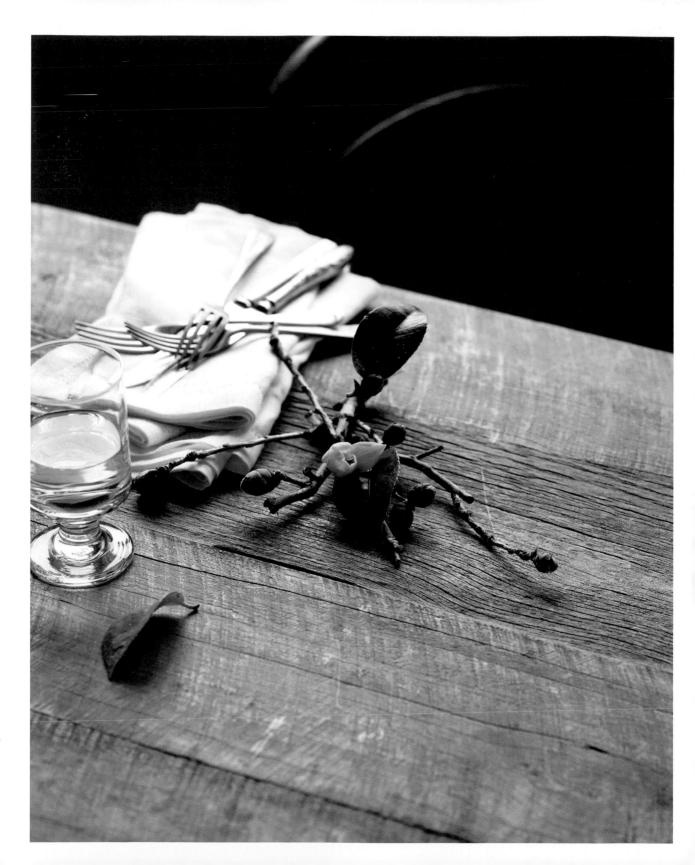

The Low-FODMAP Diet Cookbook

150 simple and delicious recipes to relieve
symptoms of IBS, Crohn's disease, coeliac disease
and other digestive disorders

SUE SHEPHERD, PhD

Vermilion
LONDON

10 9 8 7 6 5 4 3 2 1

Vermilion, an imprint of Ebury Publishing
20 Vauxhall Bridge Road,
London SW1V 2SA

Ebury Publishing is part of the Penguin Random House group of companies whose addresses can
be found at global.penguinrandomhouse.com

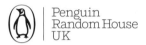

Copyright © Sue Shepherd 2013, 2014
Photographs copyright © Cath Muscat 2013

Sue Shepherd has asserted her right to be identified as the author of this Work in accordance with
the Copyright, Designs and Patents Act 1988

First published in the United Kingdom by Vermilion in 2015
First published in the United States by The Experiment, LLC in 2014
First published in Australia in 2013 as *Low FODMAP Recipes* by Viking, an imprint of Penguin Books

www.eburypublishing.co.uk

A CIP catalogue record for this book is available from the British Library

ISBN 9780091955342

Printed and bound in China by Toppan Leefung

Penguin Random House is committed to a sustainable future for our business, our readers and our
planet. This book is made from Forest Stewardship Council® certified paper.

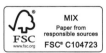

The information in this book has been compiled by way of general guidance in relation to the
specific subjects addressed, but is not a substitute and not to be relied on for medical, health-
care, pharmaceutical or other professional advice on specific circumstances and in specific
locations. So far as the author is aware the information given is correct and up to date as at
January 2015. Practice, laws and regulations all change, and the reader should obtain up to date
professional advice on any such issues. The author and publishers disclaim, as far as the law
allows, any liability arising directly or indirectly from the use, or misuse, of the information
contained in this book.

CONTENTS

Dips and Sauces

Soups & Salads

MAINS

Pasta & Rice

Ice Cream, Puddings & Custards

Tarts & Cakes

The
Low-FODMAP Diet
Cookbook

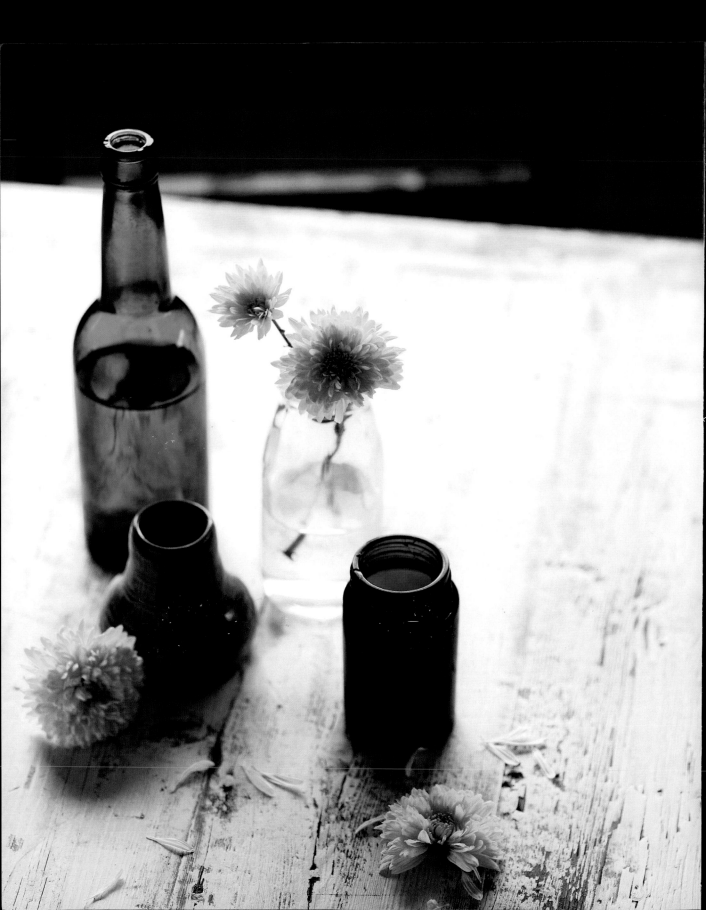

INTRODUCTION

DO YOU SUFFER FROM symptoms of irritable bowel syndrome (IBS) or another chronic digestive condition? Do you hate the idea of eating a bland diet of 'safe' foods to manage your condition, or struggle to pinpoint which foods cause your symptoms at all? Have you read and cooked from *The Complete Low-FODMAP Diet* and are you hoping for more variety in your diet?

If your answer to any of these questions is 'yes,' I am so thrilled to introduce this collection of recipes to you. Each recipe is developed specifically for those following a low-FODMAP diet. If you have not yet heard of it, FODMAP is an acronym for fermentable oligosaccharides, disaccharides, monosaccharides and polyols – you see why we had to abbreviate it! This mouthful of a term simply refers to certain carbs that ferment in your gut, releasing gas that can trigger IBS symptoms or other digestive distress. For further explanation, please see 'FODMAPs explained' (page 3).

Prior to my developing the low-FODMAP diet in 1999, there was no proven-effective treatment for irritable bowel syndrome. Clinical studies now indicate that over 75 per cent of people with IBS, many of whom have suffered for years, find relief from reducing their intake of FODMAPs. Because of this, it

has become the most recommended dietary therapy for irritable bowel syndrome (IBS), an achievement of which I am immensely proud.

I have been making these recipes for several years, as have many readers of my bestselling self-published cookbooks. These recipes were previously unavailable through UK retailers. Additionally, as our knowledge of the FODMAP content of foods has evolved over the past few years, I have tweaked the recipes to ensure they are up to date with the latest research, and as delicious as ever. I am pleased to present them to you now.

These recipes cater to those with intolerances to FODMAPs – including fructose, lactose, sorbitol, fructans and galacto-oligosaccharides. They have been developed for good health and great flavour, making it easy for the whole family to sit down and enjoy a meal together. The recipes range from simple to more complex, so they will appeal to both the novice and the more experienced cook.

The recipes are not only suitable for people following a low-FODMAP diet; they are also ideal for those on a gluten-free diet. Having coeliac disease myself, I know firsthand how important it is to make gluten-free food tempting and delicious so that nobody feels like they are missing out.

Every recipe is low-FODMAP and gluten-free, with options and substitutions for those following vegetarian or vegan, low-carb, low-fat and dairy-free diets.

Best wishes for good health always, and enjoy!

Dr Sue Shepherd

FODMAPS EXPLAINED

Irritable bowel syndrome

Irritable bowel syndrome (IBS) is a condition that affects approximately 15 per cent of the population. It affects males and females of all ages. Symptoms include excess flatulence; abdominal bloating, distension, pain or discomfort; and altered bowel habits (diarrhoea, constipation or a combination of both). These symptoms fluctuate in their severity from day to day and week to week.

Because the diagnosis of IBS is based on the pattern of the symptoms, it is important to rule out other conditions that have the same symptoms, such as coeliac disease and inflammatory bowel disease (IBD), both of which can mimic IBS. Anyone with symptoms of IBS should be examined for these disorders *before* going on a low-FODMAP or gluten-free diet, so speak with your doctor about being tested if you haven't already (see page 5 for more information). However, bear in mind that is possible to have both IBS and another digestive disorder.

The low-FODMAP diet

I developed the low-FODMAP diet in 1999, and it has been shown to help at least three out of four people with IBS, a condition that has been difficult to manage in the past. It also shows promise for treating persistent symptoms associated with coeliac disease, Crohn's disease and ulcerative colitis.

I have included a summary of the diet's principles below, but more in-depth information is available in *The Complete Low-FODMAP Diet*, which I coauthored. Please also consult with a doctor and registered dietitian before embarking on a low-FODMAP diet.

FODMAPs are a group of naturally occurring sugars that are not absorbed in the small intestine; instead, they travel down the rest of the digestive tract and arrive into the large intestine, where bacteria are present (which is normal and healthy). These bacteria use the unabsorbed sugars (FODMAPs) as a food source. When the bacteria munch on the FODMAPs, they ferment them, and this results in the release of gas, which can lead to excessive flatulence, gassiness, bloating and abdominal distension and pain. The FODMAPs can also change how quickly the bowels work, so can lead to constipation or diarrhoea (or a combination of both) in susceptible people. So it is very clear how FODMAPs trigger symptoms of IBS.

All the recipes in this book use ingredients that are low in FODMAPs – that is, they exclude the ingredients known to be high in FODMAPs (see table on page 8).

FODMAP is an acronym that stands for:

FERMENTABLE

- These poorly absorbed sugars are fermented by bacteria in the large intestine (bowel).

OLIGOSACCHARIDES

- *Oligo* means few, and *saccharide* means sugar. So these are individual sugars, joined together to make a chain.
- The two main oligosaccharides that are FODMAPs are:
  - ➤ **Fructans,** made up of fructose sugars joined together to make a chain (with glucose at the very end).
  - ➤ **Galacto-oligosaccharides** (GOS), made up of galactose sugars joined together, with a fructose and glucose at the very end.

DISACCHARIDES

- *Di* means two, and *saccharide* means sugar. So these are two individual sugars, joined together to make a double sugar.
- The important FODMAP disaccharide is lactose, made up of an individual glucose sugar joined to an individual galactose sugar.

MONOSACCHARIDES

- *Mono* means one, and *saccharide* means sugar. So these are individual sugars.
- The important FODMAP monosaccharide is excess fructose. Not all fructose needs to be avoided. Only foods that contain more fructose than glucose (or 'excess fructose' foods) need to be avoided on the low-FODMAP diet.
- If a food contains more glucose than fructose, or if glucose and fructose are present in equal ('balanced') amounts, then it is suitable on the low-FODMAP diet.
- If a food (for example, a piece of fruit) contains more glucose than fructose, or equal amounts of fructose and glucose, it is suitable to eat; however, only one piece of suitable fruit should be consumed at a time. This doesn't mean you can only have one piece of fruit per day! You can have several, but spread them out so that you only have one per sitting.

AND POLYOLS

- A polyol is made up of a sugar molecule with an alcohol side-chain. Polyols are also known as sugar alcohols, but I promise they won't make you feel intoxicated!
- The two polyols most commonly occurring in foods are sorbitol and mannitol.

Breath testing for sugar malabsorption

Though all FODMAPs may trigger symptoms of IBS, there are breath hydrogen (or methane) tests available to determine individual sensitivity to certain sugars, especially fructose, lactose and sorbitol. Breath tests are not a prerequisite for following the low-FODMAP diet but can be helpful in planning it. Ask your doctor if you are interested in having these tests run.

The tests work on the basis that bacteria in the large intestine produce hydrogen and/or methane gas by fermenting carbohydrates. Although some of the gas produced in the large intestine is passed out as flatulence, most of it is transferred across the lining of the large intestine into the bloodstream. The gases then dissolve into the blood, and the blood carries it to the lungs, where it is breathed out and can be measured.

Different testing centres have different guidelines for breath tests; however, you generally need to follow a low-FODMAP diet the day before the test to ensure that there is no hydrogen or methane already in your breath on the day of your test. A sample of your breath is collected into a special airtight bag and is then tested for the presence of hydrogen and/or methane, measured in parts per million. This is considered your baseline breath test. You then drink a solution containing a specific sugar (e.g., fructose, lactose or sorbitol). Only one sugar can be tested at a time, and each sugar must be tested on a different day within the span of a month. Once you have drunk the solution, you breathe into a new airtight bag at regular intervals over a period of around three hours. Each testing centre has different criteria for defining malabsorption of sugars tested. It is also helpful to keep a record of any symptoms you experienced at the time of the test.

For more information on breath hydrogen testing, see www.thelowfodmapdiet.com.

Lactose intolerance

Lactose is a naturally occurring sugar that is found in cow's, goat's and sheep's milk. Typically in people with lactose intolerance, the body stops making enough lactase, the enzyme that breaks down the sugar lactose. However, people can differ in the severity of their intolerance. Most people are able to tolerate small amounts of lactose (up to 4 grams) in their diet.

Lactose intolerance can cause symptoms of IBS. Additionally, many people with coeliac disease have a secondary lactose intolerance, meaning an intolerance caused by the damage to their small intestine. Secondary lactose intolerance is generally but not always temporary.

Lactose is present in large amounts in milk, ice cream and pudding. It is present in small to moderate amounts in products such as yogurt, cream, crème fraîche and soft or unripened cheeses (e.g., cottage, ricotta and cream cheese). Hard and ripened cheeses (cheddar, Parmesan, Camembert, Edam, Gouda, blue, mozzarella, etc.) and butter are virtually free of lactose.

The majority of recipes in this book are lactose-free or contain only minimal amounts of lactose. Recipes that require modification provide suggestions.

Fructose malabsorption

Fructose malabsorption is a condition in which the small intestine is impaired in its ability to absorb fructose (a naturally occurring sugar). Fructose malabsorption is different from hereditary fructose intolerance (HFI), a condition usually diagnosed in children in which the complete inability to digest fructose may result in symptoms such as vomiting, low blood sugar and jaundice, and can lead to death.

Fortunately, in people who have fructose malabsorption, there still exists a pathway through which fructose can be absorbed in the small intestine. If glucose is present at the same time, the glucose 'piggybacks' the fructose across the intestine into the bloodstream.

This is good news for fructose malabsorbers. It means that fructose and foods that contain it do not need to be avoided altogether (as is the case with HFI).

As mentioned previously, only foods that contain more fructose than glucose (excess fructose foods) need to be avoided on the low-FODMAP diet.

If a food contains more glucose than fructose, or if glucose and fructose are present in equal amounts, then it is *suitable* on the low-FODMAP diet. However, fructose malabsorbers do need to be aware of serving sizes. Only consume one serving of suitable food (such as fruit) at a time. Spread them out through the day so you only have one per meal or sitting.

Although all the recipes have been formulated with ingredients that are suitable for fructose malabsorption, ensure that you limit the serving size of any fruit-based dish to the quantity indicated in the recipe. Consuming large quantities of even 'safe' fruits can cause symptoms.

Wheat as an ingredient

Both a gluten-free diet and a low-FODMAP diet restrict wheat. On a low-FODMAP diet, this is due to wheat's fructan content rather than its gluten content. The good news is that although wheat is a source of both fructans and gluten, not every wheat ingredient contains both (see right).

You will notice that some ingredients in the recipes are specified as 'gluten-free'. Gluten must be avoided by those with coeliac disease, and is present in wheat, rye and barley. Some people on a gluten-free diet also react to oats. Every recipe in this book is gluten-free, which also ensures that fructans from wheat, rye and barley are restricted.

If you do not need to follow a gluten-free diet, you need not seek out gluten-free-labelled versions of some ingredients, such as sauces, which are unlikely to contain enough fructans to trigger a reaction.

SUITABILITY OF WHEAT PRODUCTS

Ingredient	Suitable for gluten-free diet	Suitable for low-FODMAP diet
White wheat flour	✕	✕
Whole wheat flour	✕	✕
Wheat starch	✕	✓
Modified food starch (wheat)	✕	✓
Wheat thickener	✕	✓
Wheat maltodextrin	✕	✓
Wheat dextrin	✕	✓
Wheat dextrose	✓	✓
Wheat glucose	✓	✓
Wheat glucose syrup	✓	✓
Caramel colour (rarely from wheat in UK)	✓	✓

Coeliac disease

Coeliac disease is an auto-immune disease in which the immune system's response to gluten severely injures the body. Gluten is the main protein component of wheat, rye and barley (and some people with coeliac disease also react to avenin, a protein in oats). In people with coeliac disease, the immune response to gluten causes damage to the lining of the small intestine, particularly the villi, fingerlike structures that help absorb nutrients. As a result of dramatically decreased nutrient absorption and ongoing inflammation, people with coeliac disease may become very ill. Typical symptoms can include bloating, gas, pain, diarrhoea or constipation or a combination of both, fatigue, iron deficiency, anaemia and infertility. People with untreated coeliac disease are also at greater risk for certain cancers and other maladies.

Coeliac disease is diagnosed by antibody blood tests and a confirming endoscopic biopsy of the small intestine if the tests are positive. People being tested for coeliac disease need to be eating gluten for the tests to be useful; otherwise, false negatives are common.

Coeliac disease is a lifelong condition treated by a diet free from *all* gluten. This prevents further damage to the villi and allows them to return to normal so that nutrients can be properly absorbed.

The gluten-free diet permits fruits, vegetables, meat, fish, chicken, legumes (including lentils), most dairy foods, oils and margarines and many grains. Breads, pasta and cereals can be made from alternative sources, including corn, rice, soy, buckwheat, sorghum, nuts and legumes, to name a few. These days, there are many speciality gluten-free products available, and many of those are also low-FODMAP. Look for them in the health food section of supermarkets and in health food stores.

For people prescribed a gluten-free diet, the change in lifestyle is often overwhelming. Learning which foods are suitable and which foods are no longer permitted in the diet is time-consuming at first, and the diet can seem very restrictive. I hope that this book will help you enjoy the great tastes of a gluten-free *and* low-FODMAP diet with confidence.

While every effort has been made to indicate and ensure gluten-free and low-FODMAP ingredients, it is essential to read the ingredients list of all food products to determine whether they are suitable for inclusion in your diet. The recipes in this book comply with the FSA's gluten-free labelling standards at the time of printing and exclude foods known at the time of printing to be high in FODMAPs. However, the gluten-free status of individual brands may change, the process of testing foods for their FODMAP content is ongoing, and the finished recipes have not been laboratory tested for FODMAP levels. Gluten-free labelling standards in other countries may also be different from the FSA's, so I stress again the importance of reading *all* food labels. Always assess your own level of tolerance when it comes to specific FODMAPs and recommended serving sizes.

For more information, see www.shepherd-works.com.au.

Inflammatory bowel disease (IBD)

IBD includes Crohn's disease and ulcerative colitis, illnesses in which the bowel becomes chronically inflamed. Symptoms include diarrhoea (sometimes bloody), abdominal pain, bloating, gas and fatigue. As for coeliac disease, the 'gold standard' for diagnosing IBD is an intestinal endoscopy with biopsies, though blood tests, stool samples, colonoscopies and other medical procedures may also be considered.

The causes of IBD are not known, and treatment is directed toward controlling the inflammation and preventing it from returning. Those whose bowel inflammation is well controlled but whose gastrointestinal symptoms continue may find the low-FODMAP diet a useful tool.

FOODS KNOWN TO BE HIGH IN FODMAPS THAT SHOULD THEREFORE BE RESTRICTED*

Additives (sweeteners and added fibre)**:** fructo-oligosaccharides, high-fructose corn syrup, honey, inulin, isomalt, mannitol, maltitol, polydextrose, sorbitol, xylitol

Cereal and grain foods: bran (from wheat, rye or barley); bread (from wheat, rye or barley); breakfast cereals, granolas and muesli (from wheat, rye or barley); crackers (from wheat or rye); pasta, including couscous and gnocchi (from wheat); wheat noodles (chow mein, udon, etc.)

Drinks: chamomile and fennel tea, chicory-based coffee substitutes, juices made from unsuitable fruits (below)

Fruits: apples, apricots, Asian pears, blackberries, boysenberries, cherries, figs, mangoes, nectarines, peaches, pears, persimmons, plums, prunes, tamarillos, watermelon, white peaches

Legumes: beans (all kinds, including certain forms of soy, such as textured vegetable protein/TVP), chickpeas, lentils

Milk and milk products: custard, ice cream, milk (cow's, goat's and sheep's, including whole, semi-skimmed, skimmed, evaporated and condensed), pudding, soft cheeses, yogurt (cow's, sheep's or goat's)

Nuts: cashews, pistachios

Vegetables: artichokes (globe and Jerusalem), asparagus, cauliflower, garlic (and garlic powder in large amounts), leeks, mangetouts, mushrooms, onions (red, white, yellow and onion powder), spring onions (white part), shallots, snow peas, sugar snap peas

FOODS KNOWN TO BE MODERATE IN FODMAPS THAT SHOULD THEREFORE BE EATEN IN MODERATION

Fruits: cherries, longans, lychee, pomegranate, rambutan

Milk and milk products: cottage cheese, cream, cream cheese, crème fraîche, mascarpone, ricotta

Nuts: almonds, hazelnuts

Vegetables: avocado, beetroot, broccoli, Brussels sprouts, butternut squash, celery, corn, fennel, green peas, savoy cabbage, sweet potato

Note: Courtesy Monash University, Department of Gastroenterology

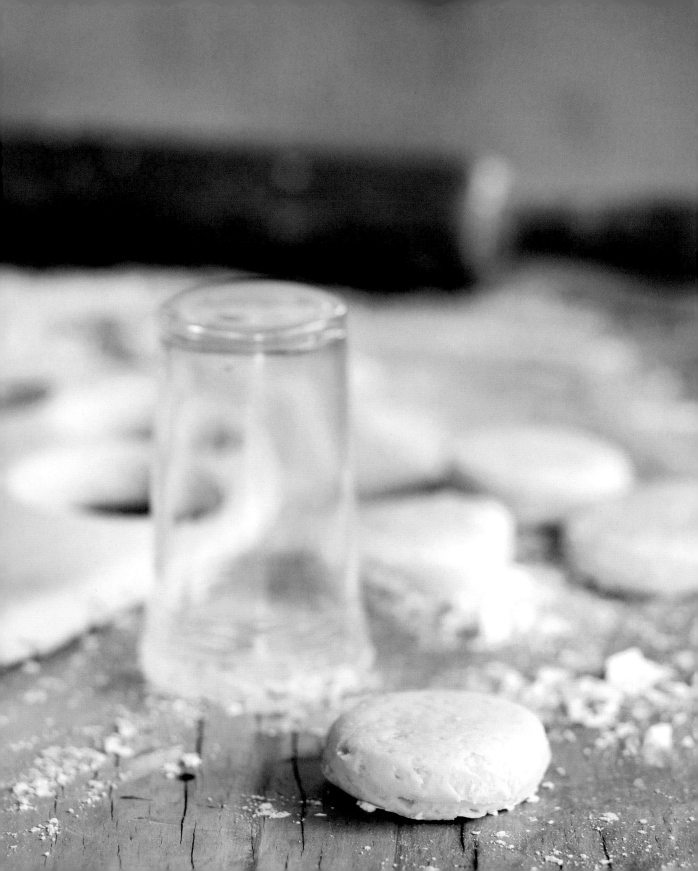

SUBSTITUTIONS

The recipes in this book are intended to be easily adaptable to many different dietary needs, not just FODMAP intolerance. Read on for some substitution suggestions.

Vegetarian and vegan

Vegetarians and vegans can eat well on a low-FODMAP diet, but it requires careful planning. A variety of plant-based proteins contain FODMAPs (such as whole wheat, barley, legumes and certain nuts and soy foods). Vegetarians and vegans who do not tolerate these FODMAPs may be at risk of not meeting their daily protein needs. If you are vegetarian, you may eat eggs and dairy foods (lactose-free or low-lactose if necessary).

Otherwise, you can be sure of meeting your protein needs by consuming nuts and seeds, suitable soy products such as tofu and tempeh, cereal products based on high-protein, low-FODMAP grains and cereals and protein-enriched milk alternatives. Provided you do not need to be gluten-free, you can also incorporate seitan (a vegan meat substitute made of vital wheat gluten) into your diet. Because it is made entirely of protein, it does not contain the problematic FODMAP carbohydrates.

To make recipes in this book vegetarian or vegan, follow specific instructions in the recipes or try these basic swaps:

- For meat or seafood: firm or extra firm tofu (pressed, if desired, for at least 15 minutes between paper towels and plates with extra weight on top); cubed or crumbled tempeh (steamed, if desired, for 10 to 20 minutes); homemade or shop-bought onion-free, garlic-free seitan (*not* gluten-free)
- For eggs: 1 tablespoon psyllium husk, ground flaxseeds or chia seeds mixed with 3 tablespoons water; commercial egg replacer; mashed banana (in some baked goods)
- For milk: soy milk made from soybean extract; unsweetened almond milk; rice milk; coconut milk
- For butter: soy-free vegan 'butter' or vegetable shortening; vegetable oil including coconut oil; nut butters or mashed banana (in baking)
- For cheese: puréed squash or sweet potato (for creaminess); crushed nuts or seeds and their butters (for taste, texture and protein); dairy-free, soy-free vegan cheese
- For yogurt: soy yogurt made from soybean extract; almond yogurt; coconut yogurt
- For gelatin: vegan gelatin; agar or carrageenan seaweed

Low-fat

Most of the recipes in this book are suitable for those following a low-fat diet, but some substitutions may be necessary. Fat can be a trigger for IBS symptoms, so you may wish to reduce your intake of fat as well as FODMAPs. Keep in mind, though, that some fat is necessary to a healthy diet. Before making changes to your diet, speak with a registered dietitian. In the recipes, try these basic swaps:

- *For meat:* white chicken or pork meat (fat trimmed); lean minced beef, pork and lamb; fish and shellfish; any of the vegetarian and vegan options outlined in the previous section
- *For eggs:* egg whites
- *For milk:* semi-skimmed or skimmed milk (lactose-free if required); soy milk made from soybean extract; almond milk
- *For butter:* margarine; low-fat soy-free buttery spreads
- *For yogurt and cheese:* low-fat varieties

If you can tolerate one or more types of FODMAPs

Keep in mind that the low-FODMAP diet is highly individualised. Although it is recommended to spend six weeks restricting all FODMAPs, most people following the diet are able to add various foods – sometimes in limited quantities – back into their diet. (See *The Complete Low-FODMAP Diet* for more details on 'challenging' foods.) The goal of the diet is not to restrict your menu to the point that you are eating bland or repetitive meals; the goal is to help you enjoy your food without gastrointestinal symptoms!

Therefore, if you have determined you are able to tolerate certain FODMAPs, there is no reason not to use foods containing them in the book's recipes. Those who can tolerate polyols, for example, may wish to add small amounts of their favourite stone fruit into certain dessert recipes; and those who can tolerate fructans may wish to buy wheat bread rather than more expensive gluten-free varieties.

BREAKFAST
&
BRUNCH

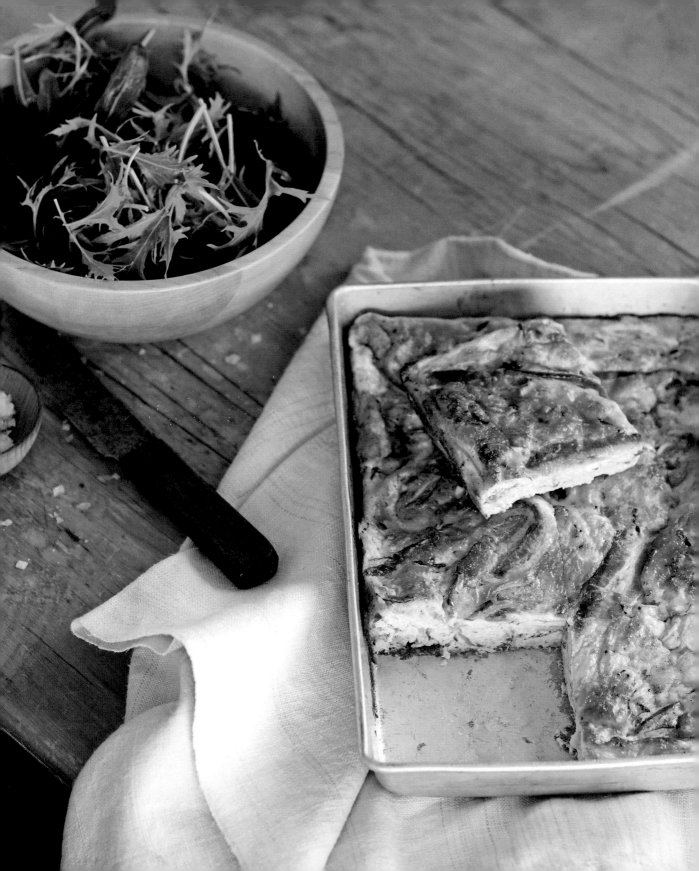

Bacon and Courgette Crustless Quiche

Serve this with a green salad for a light brunch. It's also nicely portable, so pack it in a picnic basket or school lunchbox if you want to take it on the go.

1. Preheat the oven to 170°C. Grease a 23-cm quiche dish or pie tin and line with a parchment paper circle. Line a plate with paper towels.

2. Add the bacon to an unheated frying pan and turn the heat to medium. Cook, turning occasionally, for about 10 minutes, or until crispy. Transfer to the prepared plate to drain. When the bacon is cool enough to handle, break into small pieces.

3. Combine the bacon, courgette, cheese, oil and eggs in a large bowl. Season with salt and pepper. Pour into the baking dish and bake for 20 to 25 minutes, until firm and golden brown. Remove from the oven and let stand for 5 minutes before slicing. Serve it warm or cold – it's delicious either way – with a green salad, if desired.

PER SERVING (not including the green salad): 258 calories; 16 g protein; 20 g total fat; 8 g saturated fat; 3 g carbohydrates; 1 g fibre; 665 mg sodium

10 bacon slices, at room temperature

2 large courgettes, grated

180 g grated cheddar

2 tablespoons canola oil

6 large eggs, lightly beaten

Salt and freshly ground black pepper

Green salad, for serving (optional)

Scrambled Eggs

Few things are more delicious than a plate of perfectly cooked scrambled eggs, and luckily, eggs – like other protein foods – are always welcome on a low-FODMAP diet. Enjoy this dish simply seasoned with salt and pepper, or ramp it up with a sprinkling of fresh chives (or any other herbs you like) and thinly sliced sautéed veggies or smoked salmon.

10 large eggs

180 ml lactose-free milk

Salt and freshly ground black pepper

45 g salted butter

Toasted gluten-free, soy-free bread, for serving

1. Crack the eggs into a large bowl, add the milk and whisk until combined. Season with salt and pepper.
2. Melt the butter in a medium frying pan over low heat. Pour in the egg mixture. Use a wooden spoon to gently push the egg mixture from the edge into the middle of the pan to prevent sticking. Cook for 4 to 5 minutes, continuing to gently stir, until nearly cooked – the eggs should still be creamy and slightly runny. Serve immediately with toasted gluten-free bread.

PER SERVING (not including the toast): 282 calories; 17 g protein; 22 g total fat; 10 g saturated fat; 4 g carbohydrates; 0 g fibre; 560 mg sodium

Omelette Wraps

MAKES 6

If you used to enjoy pita wraps, then this is a perfect alternative. You can fill them with anything you like, such as this autumn-inspired mix. Another quick and easy way to make super-thin omelettes is to spray a panini press with non-stick cooking spray, add a beaten egg, lower the lid and cook for 30 seconds. Done!

1. Place a medium non-stick frying pan over medium heat and spray with cooking spray. Crack an egg into a small bowl and whisk with a fork. Pour the egg into the hot pan and tilt to coat the bottom – you want the omelette to be about 12 cm in diameter. Cook for 30 to 60 seconds, then flip with a spatula or pancake turner, taking care not to tear the omelette. Cook for 30 to 60 seconds more, then carefully remove from the pan and set aside on a plate. Repeat with the remaining eggs to make 6 omelettes. Set aside to cool.

2. To assemble, place an omelette on a flat surface. Lay a slice of turkey breast down the centre of the omelette and top with ½ teaspoon cranberry sauce, a few slices of avocado (if using) and tomato, baby spinach leaves and a sprinkling of carrot. Fold the bottom third of the omelette toward the centre, then fold in the left and right sides to encase the filling (almost as if you were rolling a burrito). Repeat with the remaining omelettes and filling. Serve immediately, or cover and refrigerate until you're ready to eat.

PER SERVING (including the avocado): 159 calories; 11 g protein; 10 g total fat; 3 g saturated fat; 6 g carbohydrates; 2 g fibre; 85 mg sodium

Non-stick cooking spray

6 large eggs

6 thin slices cooked turkey breast (about 100 g)

1 heaped tablespoon cranberry sauce

1 avocado, pitted, peeled and sliced (optional)

1 tomato, sliced

2 handfuls of baby spinach leaves, rinsed and dried

60 g grated carrot (1 medium)

Light Omelette with Chicken and Spinach

SERVES 2

This is perfect for breakfast, lunch or dinner, and a really great way to use up leftover roast chicken (such as Soy-Infused Roast Chicken, page 135). Alternatively, you can use cubed tofu or gluten-free ham, shredded turkey, pieces of seitan and/or additional suitable veggies.

1. Whisk together the eggs, basil and parsley in a medium bowl. Season with salt and pepper.

2. Heat the oil in a medium frying pan over medium heat. Add the egg mixture and tilt to coat the bottom of the pan. Cook until almost set on top. Using a spatula or pancake turner, carefully lift the edges and shake the omelette loose.

3. Scatter the chicken, spinach, pepper and cheese over one half of the omelette. Fold the other half over the top to cover the filling. Cook briefly until the filling is heated through and the cheese is starting to melt. Slide the omelette out of the pan and cut it in half (or just serve whole with two forks!). If preferred, you can split the ingredients in half and make 2 smaller omelettes.

4 large eggs

5 g roughly chopped basil

15 g roughly chopped flat-leaf parsley

Salt and freshly ground black pepper

1 tablespoon canola oil

80 g shredded cooked chicken

Small handful of baby spinach leaves, rinsed, dried and chopped

½ red pepper, diced

30 g grated cheddar

PER SERVING: 343 calories; 29 g protein; 23 g total fat; 7 g saturated fat; 4 g carbohydrates; 1 g fibre; 542 mg sodium

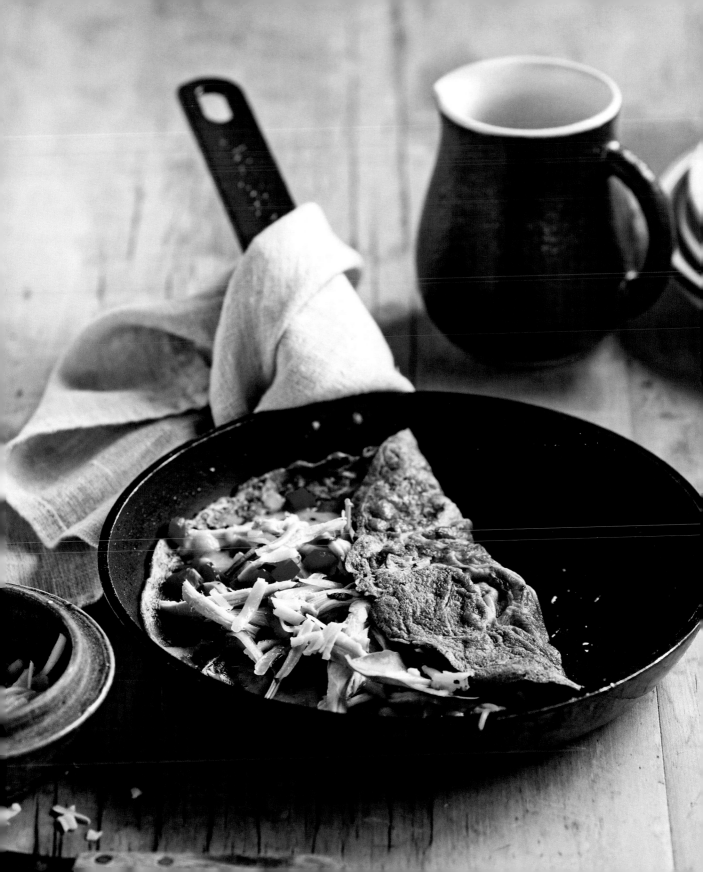

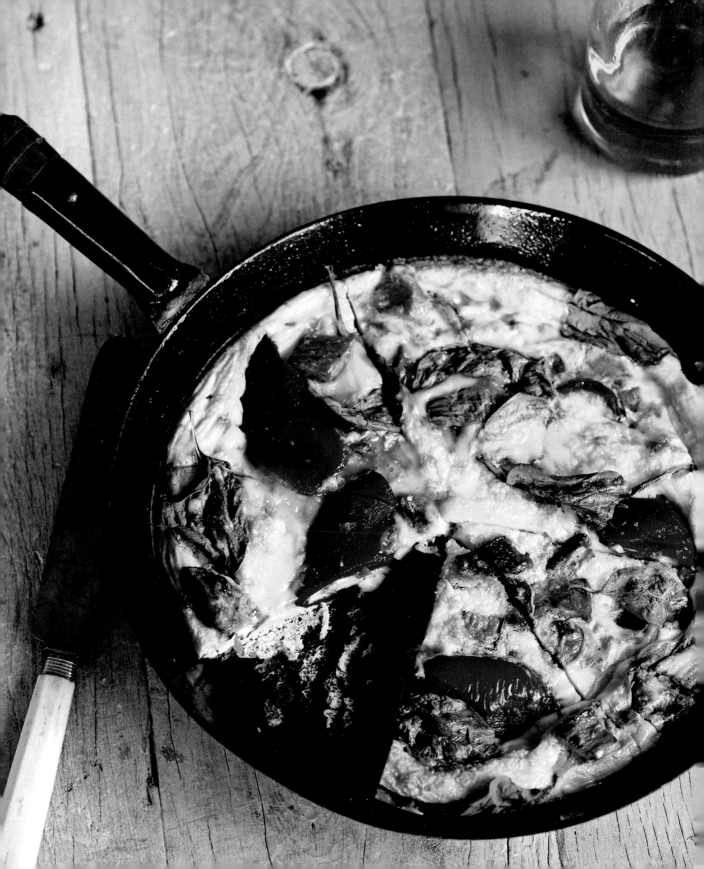

Roasted Sweet Potato and Red Pepper Frittata

SERVES 6–8

This is one of my favourite flavour combinations for a frittata, but of course you can use other low-FODMAP vegetables if you prefer. Serve it with a fresh green salad.

1. Preheat the oven to 180°C.

2. Place the sweet potato and peppers in a glass baking dish, drizzle with a little olive oil and bake for 10 to 15 minutes, until golden brown and tender. Remove from the oven, wrap in foil and let cool. Leave the oven on.

3. Peel the cooled peppers and discard the skins. Cut the peppers into large pieces.

4. Grease a 23-cm ovenproof frying pan. Line the bottom with a layer of sweet potato and top with a layer of peppers. Sprinkle with some of the spinach leaves. Continue with the remaining vegetables, finishing with a layer of peppers.

5. Lightly beat the eggs in a bowl and season with salt and pepper. Pour the eggs over the vegetables and gently tilt the dish to make sure they are evenly distributed and fill all the gaps.

6. Bake for 20 to 30 minutes, until firm when touched in the middle. Remove from the oven and let rest for 5 minutes before cutting. Serve warm or cold.

1 large sweet potato, peeled (if desired) and chopped

2 red peppers, seeded and cut into quarters

Olive oil, for drizzling and greasing the pan

1 large handful of baby spinach leaves, rinsed and dried

10 large eggs

Salt and freshly ground black pepper

PER SERVING (⅛ recipe): 140 calories; 8 g protein; 8 g total fat; 2 g saturated fat; 8 g carbohydrates; 1 g fibre; 229 mg sodium

Cheese and Herb Scones

MAKES 10–12

These can be made with any herbs you like. They are great to have on hand for a weekend brunch or afterschool snack, and they also make a delicious accompaniment to homemade soup.

1. Preheat the oven to 200°C. Line a baking sheet with parchment paper.

2. Whisk the milk and egg in a bowl. Stir in the Parmesan, cheddar and herbs.

3. Sift the cornflour, tapioca flour, soy flour, xanthan gum and baking powder three times into a medium bowl (or whisk in the bowl until well combined). Rub in the butter with your fingertips until the mixture resembles fine breadcrumbs. Add the milk mixture all at once and mix with a large metal spoon until the dough begins to hold together.

4. Lightly sprinkle your work surface with cornflour. Gently bring the dough together with your hands and turn out onto the floured surface. Knead gently by pressing and then turning until the dough is just smooth (use a light touch or the scones will be tough).

5. Using a lightly floured rolling pin, roll out the dough to a thickness of 2.5 cm and cut out 10 to 12 scones with a 5-cm biscuit or cookie cutter. Use a straight-down motion to do this (if you twist the cutter, the scones will rise unevenly during baking). It's a good idea to dip the cutter in cornflour before each cut to prevent sticking.

6. Place the scones on the sheet about 1 cm apart and brush the tops with milk. Bake for 10 to 12 minutes, until golden and cooked through. Remove the scones from the oven and immediately wrap them in a clean tea towel (this will help give them a soft crust). Serve warm.

175 ml semi-skimmed milk, lactose-free milk or suitable plant-based milk, plus more for brushing

1 large egg

40 g grated Parmesan

60 g grated cheddar

3 to 4 heaped tablespoons chopped herbs (such as oregano, thyme and flat-leaf parsley)

150 g cornflour, plus more for kneading

125 g tapioca flour

45 g soy flour

1 teaspoon xanthan gum or guar gum

2 teaspoons gluten-free baking powder

75 g unsalted butter, cut into cubes, at room temperature

PER SERVING ($\frac{1}{12}$ **recipe**): 179 calories; 6 g protein; 9 g total fat; 5 g saturated fat; 20 g carbohydrates; 1 g fibre; 172 mg sodium

Chocolate Scones

I developed this recipe for my mum. She was diagnosed with coeliac disease a few years after me, and one of the things she missed most was light, old-fashioned scones. Whether or not scones top your list of cravings, too, you can enjoy this simple addition to your breakfast, brunch and snack repertoire.

1. Preheat the oven to 200°C. Line a baking sheet with parchment paper.

2. Whisk the milk and egg in a bowl.

3. Sift the cornflour, tapioca flour, soy flour, cocoa, xanthan gum, baking powder and sugar three times into a medium bowl (or whisk in the bowl until well combined). Rub in the butter with your fingertips until the mixture resembles fine breadcrumbs. Add the chocolate chips and mix. Add the milk and egg mixture all at once and mix with a large metal spoon until the dough begins to hold together.

4. Lightly sprinkle your work surface with cornflour. Gently bring the dough together with your hands and turn out onto the floured surface. Knead gently by pressing and then turning until the dough is just smooth (use a light touch, or the scones will be tough).

5. Using a lightly floured rolling pin, roll out the dough to a thickness of 2.5 cm and cut out 10 to 12 scones using a 5-cm biscuit or cookie cutter. Use a straight-down motion to do this (if you twist the cutter, the scones will rise unevenly during baking). It's a good idea to dip the cutter in cornflour before each cut to prevent sticking.

6. Place the scones on the sheet about 1 cm apart and brush the tops with milk. Bake for 10 to 12 minutes, until golden and cooked through. Remove the scones from the oven and immediately wrap them in a clean tea towel (this will help give them a soft crust). Serve warm with jam and butter.

PER SERVING (¹⁄₁₂ **recipe**): 175 calories; 3 g protein; 8 g total fat; 4 g saturated fat; 26 g carbohydrates; 2 g fibre; 73 mg sodium

150 ml semi-skimmed milk, lactose-free milk or suitable plant-based milk, plus more for kneading

1 large egg

150 g cornflour, plus more for dusting

125 g tapioca flour

45 g soy flour

2 heaped tablespoons cocoa

1 teaspoon xanthan gum or guar gum

1¾ teaspoons gluten-free baking powder

55 g caster sugar

75 g unsalted butter, cut into cubes, at room temperature

90 g chocolate chips*

Jam or butter, for serving

---

* Most chocolate chips are low-FODMAP, but check the labels and avoid high-fructose corn syrup. If you follow a gluten-free diet, confirm that the brand is gluten-free.

Blueberry Pancakes

SERVES 4–6

These pancakes are one of the best Sunday brunches you can serve, but I must confess I find them hard to resist at any time of the day. Frozen blueberries work just as well as fresh, so you can enjoy this breakfast all year round. Look for xanthan gum, an important binding agent, in health food shops or the health food section of your local supermarket. As an alternative, you may use guar gum.

1. Whisk together the eggs and milk in a small bowl or liquid measuring cup.

2. Sift the rice flour, cornflour, soy flour, brown sugar, baking powder and xanthan gum three times into a large bowl (or whisk in the bowl until well combined). Make a well in the centre and gradually pour in the milk mixture, mixing well to make a smooth batter. Stir in the melted butter, cover and set aside for 15 minutes.

3. Heat a large non-stick frying pan or griddle over medium heat and spray with cooking spray. Working in batches, pour in enough batter to form 10-cm pancakes (125 ml each) and cook for 1 minute or until they start to set. Sprinkle 8 blueberries onto each pancake and cook for 2 minutes more. Turn and cook for 2 minutes or until cooked through. Transfer to a plate and cover loosely with foil to keep warm. Repeat with the remaining batter and berries to make 12 pancakes in total.

4. Sprinkle with the remaining blueberries and serve immediately with maple syrup (if desired) and/or whipped cream for an especially decadent treat.

PER SERVING (⅙ recipe, not including syrup or cream): 385 calories; 9 g protein; 12 g total fat; 6 g saturated fat; 61 g carbohydrates; 2 g fibre; 396 mg sodium

2 large eggs

375 ml semi-skimmed milk, lactose-free milk or suitable plant-based milk

130 g superfine white rice flour

75 g cornflour

45 g soy flour

150 g packed light brown sugar

1 tablespoon plus 1 teaspoon gluten-free baking powder

1 teaspoon xanthan gum or guar gum

60 g salted butter, melted

Non-stick cooking spray

150 g fresh or frozen blueberries

Maple syrup and/or whipped cream, for serving (optional)

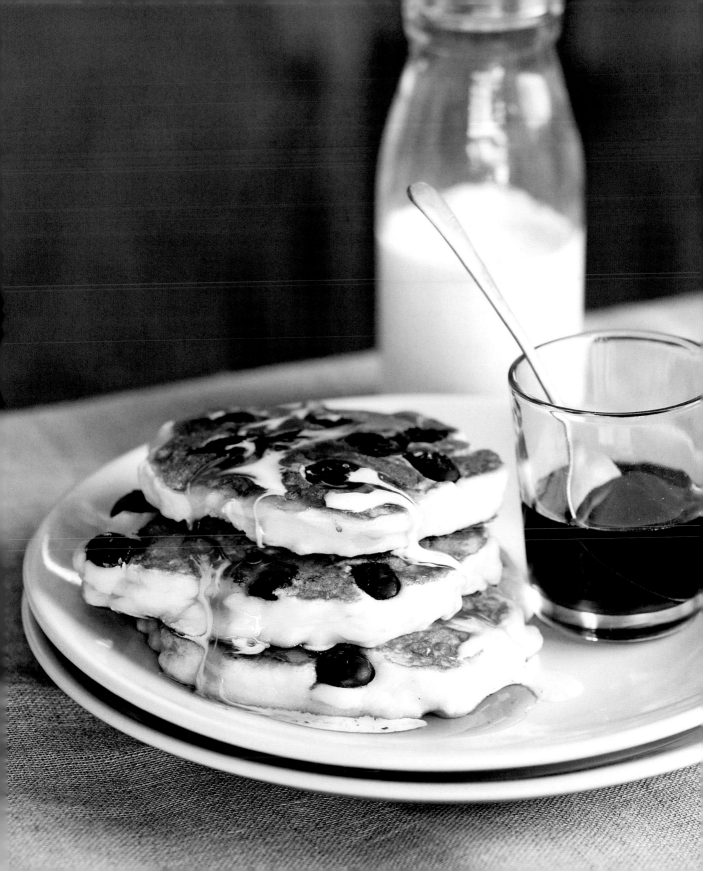

MUFFINS

EACH RECIPE MAKES 12

Muffins are the perfect lunchbox treat. They also freeze well – just cook up a batch and eat one (or two) first, then store them in an airtight bag or container in the freezer. Of course, the great thing about muffins is their versatility: you can use virtually any ingredients you like. I have given a few suggestions for both sweet and savoury muffins over the next couple of pages.

Pumpkin Muffins

130 g superfine white rice flour
75 g cornflour
90 g potato flour
2 teaspoons gluten-free baking powder
1 teaspoon baking soda
1 teaspoon xanthan gum or guar gum
2 teaspoons pumpkin pie spice
1 heaped tablespoon ground cinnamon
45 g unsalted butter, melted
200 g gluten-free low-fat vanilla yogurt
2 large eggs
400 g mashed cooked pumpkin, kabocha or other suitable winter squash
   (from about 500 g peeled and seeded raw squash)
220 g caster sugar

1. Preheat the oven to 170°C and line a 12-cup muffin tin with paper liners.
2. Sift the rice flour, cornflour, potato flour, baking powder, baking soda, xanthan gum, pumpkin pie spice and cinnamon three times into a large bowl (or whisk in the bowl until well combined).
3. Combine the melted butter, yogurt and eggs in a medium bowl. Stir in the squash and sugar. Add to the flour mixture and stir with a large metal spoon until just combined (do not overmix). Pour the batter evenly into the muffin cups until they are two-thirds full.
4. Bake for 15 to 20 minutes, until golden brown and a toothpick inserted into the centre of a muffin comes out clean. Cool in the pan for 5 minutes, then turn out onto a wire rack to cool completely.

PER SERVING: 209 calories; 3 g protein; 4 g total fat; 2 g saturated fat; 41 g carbohydrates; 2 g fibre; 196 mg sodium

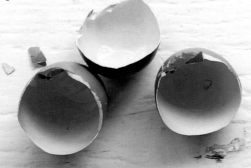

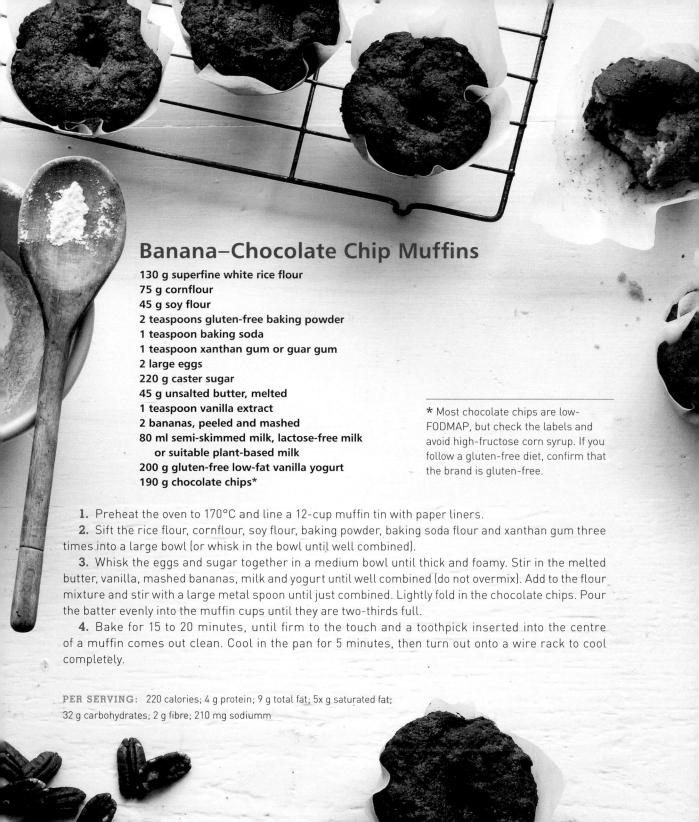

Banana–Chocolate Chip Muffins

130 g superfine white rice flour
75 g cornflour
45 g soy flour
2 teaspoons gluten-free baking powder
1 teaspoon baking soda
1 teaspoon xanthan gum or guar gum
2 large eggs
220 g caster sugar
45 g unsalted butter, melted
1 teaspoon vanilla extract
2 bananas, peeled and mashed
80 ml semi-skimmed milk, lactose-free milk
    or suitable plant-based milk
200 g gluten-free low-fat vanilla yogurt
190 g chocolate chips*

* Most chocolate chips are low-FODMAP, but check the labels and avoid high-fructose corn syrup. If you follow a gluten-free diet, confirm that the brand is gluten-free.

1. Preheat the oven to 170°C and line a 12-cup muffin tin with paper liners.

2. Sift the rice flour, cornflour, soy flour, baking powder, baking soda flour and xanthan gum three times into a large bowl (or whisk in the bowl until well combined).

3. Whisk the eggs and sugar together in a medium bowl until thick and foamy. Stir in the melted butter, vanilla, mashed bananas, milk and yogurt until well combined (do not overmix). Add to the flour mixture and stir with a large metal spoon until just combined. Lightly fold in the chocolate chips. Pour the batter evenly into the muffin cups until they are two-thirds full.

4. Bake for 15 to 20 minutes, until firm to the touch and a toothpick inserted into the centre of a muffin comes out clean. Cool in the pan for 5 minutes, then turn out onto a wire rack to cool completely.

PER SERVING: 220 calories; 4 g protein; 9 g total fat; 5x g saturated fat; 32 g carbohydrates; 2 g fibre; 210 mg sodiumm

Vanilla-Rhubarb Muffins

150 g finely chopped rhubarb
330 g caster sugar
130 g superfine white rice flour
65 g tapioca flour
75 g cornflour
2 teaspoons gluten-free baking powder
1 teaspoon baking soda
1 teaspoon xanthan gum or guar gum
45 g unsalted butter, melted
½ teaspoon vanilla extract
200 g gluten-free low-fat vanilla yogurt
2 large eggs

1. Combine the rhubarb and 55 g of the sugar in a small saucepan and cover with water. Bring to a boil over high heat, reduce heat to medium and cook gently for 10 minutes or until tender. Drain and set aside to cool.

2. Preheat the oven to 170°C and line a 12-cup muffin tin with paper liners.

3. Sift the rice flour, tapioca flour, cornflour, baking powder, baking soda and xanthan gum three times into a large bowl (or whisk in the bowl until well combined).

4. Combine the melted butter, vanilla, yogurt, eggs and the remaining 275 g sugar in a medium bowl. Add the yogurt mixture to the flour mixture and stir with a large metal spoon until just combined. Do not overmix. Gently stir in the cooked rhubarb (take care, because you want the pieces to remain intact). Pour the batter evenly into the muffin cups until they are two-thirds full.

5. Bake for 12 to 15 minutes, until golden brown and a toothpick inserted into the centre of a muffin comes out clean. Cool in the pan for 5 minutes, then turn out onto a wire rack to cool completely.

PER SERVING: 221 calories; 2 g protein; 4 g total fat; 2 g saturated fat; 45 g carbohydrates; 1 g fibre; 193 mg sodium

Ginger and Pecan Muffins

130 g superfine white rice flour
65 g tapioca flour
75 g cornflour
2 teaspoons gluten-free baking powder
1 teaspoon baking soda
1 teaspoon xanthan gum or guar gum
45 g unsalted butter, melted
200 g gluten-free low-fat vanilla yogurt
2 large eggs
275 g caster sugar
60 g roughly chopped pecans
110 g chopped crystallised ginger, plus 12 small
    pieces for garnish

1. Preheat the oven to 170°C and line a 12-cup muffin tin with paper liners.

2. Sift the rice flour, tapioca flour, cornflour, baking powder, baking soda and xanthan gum three times into a large bowl (or whisk in the bowl until well combined).

3. Combine the melted butter, yogurt, eggs, sugar, pecans and ginger in a medium bowl. Add to the flour mixture and stir with a large metal spoon until just combined (do not overmix). Pour the batter evenly into the muffin cups until they are two-thirds full and top each muffin with a piece of crystallised ginger.

4. Bake for 15 to 20 minutes, until golden brown and a toothpick inserted into the centre of a muffin comes out clean. Cool in the pan for 5 minutes, then turn out onto a wire rack to cool completely.

PER SERVING: 277 calories; 3 g protein; 8 g total fat; 2 g saturated fat; 52 g carbohydrates; 1 g fibre; 197 mg sodium

Cheesy Corn Muffins

130 g superfine white rice flour
75 g cornflour
65 g tapioca flour
2 teaspoons gluten-free baking powder
1 teaspoon baking soda
1 teaspoon xanthan gum or guar gum
45 g salted butter, melted
200 g gluten-free low-fat plain yogurt
3 large eggs
60 g grated cheddar, plus twelve 1 cm cubes
40 g finely grated Parmesan
4 to 6 lean bacon slices (115 g), cooked until crispy
　　(see page 15) and crumbled (optional)
200 g drained tinned or thawed frozen corn kernels
Pinch of salt and freshly ground black pepper

1. Preheat the oven to 170°C and line a 12-cup muffin tin with paper liners.

2. Sift the rice flour, cornflour, tapioca flour, baking powder, baking soda and xanthan gum three times into a large bowl (or whisk in the bowl until well combined).

3. Combine the melted butter, yogurt, eggs, cheddar, Parmesan, bacon (if using) and corn in a medium bowl. Add the yogurt mixture to the flour mixture and stir with a large metal spoon until just combined (do not overmix). Season with salt and pepper. Half-fill the muffin cups with the batter, then place a cube of cheddar in each one. Pour in the remaining batter until the cups are two-thirds full.

4. Bake for 15 to 20 minutes, until firm to the touch and a toothpick inserted into the centre of a muffin (avoid the cheese filling) comes out clean. Cool in the pan for 5 minutes, then turn out onto a wire rack to cool completely.

PER SERVING: 218 calories; 9 g protein; 11 g total fat; 5 g saturated fat; 21 g carbohydrates; 1 g fibre; 546 mg sodium

Spinach and Tomato Muffins

130 g superfine white rice flour
75 g cornflour
45 g soy flour
2 teaspoons gluten-free baking powder
1 teaspoon baking soda
1 teaspoon xanthan gum or guar gum
75 g salted butter, melted
200 g gluten-free low-fat plain yogurt
3 large eggs
250 ml semi-skimmed milk, lactose-free milk or
　　suitable plant-based milk
100 g finely grated Parmesan
2 medium tomatoes, diced
60 g baby spinach leaves, rinsed, dried and roughly
　　chopped
Pinch of salt and freshly ground black pepper

1. Preheat the oven to 170°C and line a 12-cup muffin tin with paper liners.

2. Sift the rice flour, cornflour, soy flour, baking powder, baking soda and xanthan gum three times into a large bowl (or whisk in the bowl until well combined).

3. Combine the melted butter, yogurt, eggs, milk, Parmesan, tomatoes, spinach and salt and pepper in a medium bowl. Add to the flour mixture and mix with a wooden spoon until just combined. Pour the batter evenly into the muffin cups until they are two-thirds full.

4. Bake for 15 to 20 minutes, until firm to the touch and a toothpick inserted into the centre of a muffin comes out clean. Cool in the pan for 5 minutes, then turn out onto a wire rack to cool completely.

PER SERVING: 200 calories; 9 g protein; 10 g total fat; 5 g saturated fat; 19 g carbohydrates; 2 g fibre; 469 mg sodium

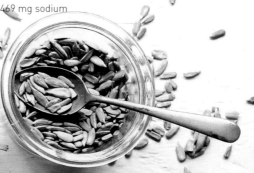

High-Fibre Muffins with Courgette and Sunflower Seeds

140 g brown rice flour
75 g cornflour
45 g soy flour
2 teaspoons gluten-free baking powder
1 teaspoon baking soda
1 teaspoon xanthan gum or guar gum
75 g salted butter, melted
125 ml semi-skimmed milk, lactose-free milk or suitable plant-based milk
200 g gluten-free low-fat plain yogurt
3 large eggs
60 g finely grated Parmesan
½ medium courgette, grated
75 g roasted unsalted sunflower seeds
60 g rice bran
25 g walnuts, crushed
¼ teaspoon freshly grated nutmeg
Pinch of salt and freshly ground black pepper

1. Preheat the oven to 170°C and line a 12-cup muffin tin with paper liners.

2. Sift the rice flour, cornflour, soy flour, baking powder, baking soda and xanthan gum three times into a large bowl (or whisk in the bowl until well combined).

3. Combine the melted butter, milk, yogurt, eggs, Parmesan, courgette, sunflower seeds, rice bran, walnuts, nutmeg and salt and pepper in a medium bowl and mix well. Add the flour mixture and mix with a wooden spoon for 2 to 3 minutes (be careful not to overmix). Pour the batter evenly into the muffin cups until they are two-thirds full.

4. Bake for 15 to 20 minutes, until firm to the touch and a toothpick inserted into the centre of a muffin comes out clean. Cool in the pan for 5 minutes, then turn out onto a wire rack to cool completely.

PER SERVING: 243 calories; 9 g protein; 14 g total fat; 5 g saturated fat; 22 g carbohydrates; 3 g fibre; 368 mg sodium

Chilli-Cheese Muffins

130 g superfine white rice flour
75 g cornflour
45 g soy flour
2 teaspoons gluten-free baking powder
1 teaspoon baking soda
1 teaspoon xanthan gum or guar gum
1 teaspoon chilli powder
75 g salted butter, melted
200 g gluten-free low-fat plain yogurt
3 large eggs
185 ml semi-skimmed milk, lactose-free milk or suitable plant-based milk
60 g finely grated Parmesan
120 g grated cheddar
2 heaped tablespoons finely chopped flat-leaf parsley
Pinch of salt and freshly ground black pepper

1. Preheat the oven to 170°C and line a 12-cup muffin tin with paper liners.

2. Sift the rice flour, cornflour, soy flour, baking powder, baking soda, xanthan gum and chilli powder three times into a large bowl (or whisk in the bowl until well combined).

3. Combine the melted butter, yogurt, eggs, milk, Parmesan, cheddar, parsley and salt and pepper in a medium bowl and mix well. Add to the flour mixture and stir with a large metal spoon until just combined. Pour the batter evenly into the muffin cups until they are two-thirds full.

4. Bake for 15 to 20 minutes, until firm to the touch and a toothpick inserted into the centre of a muffin comes out clean. Cool in the pan for 5 minutes, then turn out onto a wire rack to cool completely.

PER SERVING: 184 calories; 8 g protein; 13 g total fat; 6 g saturated fat; 13 g carbohydrates; 1 g fibre; 374 mg sodium

STARTERS & LIGHT MEALS

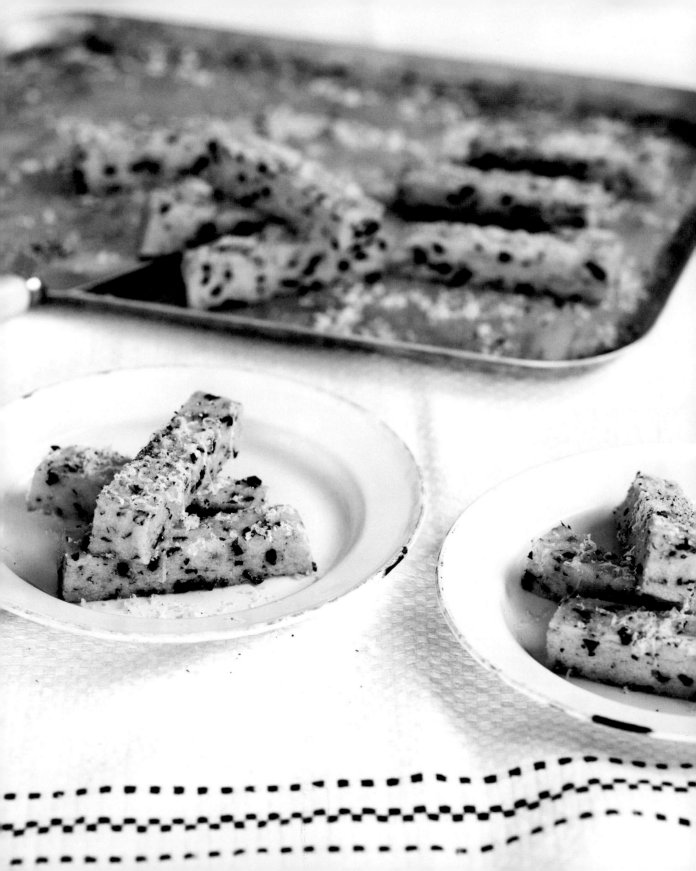

Cheese and Olive Polenta Fingers

MAKES ABOUT 30

Polenta is such a versatile food, and perfect for the low-FODMAP diet. It can be creamy (as in the Baked Atlantic Salmon on Soft Blue Cheese Polenta recipe on page 122) or firm, as in this recipe, so it can be easily cut into tasty bites.

1. Line an 20-cm square baking dish with parchment paper.

2. Pour the stock into a medium saucepan and bring to a boil. Add the cornmeal and cook over medium heat for 3 to 5 minutes, stirring constantly. By now, the polenta should be very thick. Add the olives, butter, parsley and half the Parmesan and stir until the butter and cheese have melted. Season to taste with the black pepper.

3. Pour the polenta into the baking dish and smooth the surface. Let cool slightly, then refrigerate for 1 hour.

4. Preheat the oven to 180°C and line a baking sheet with parchment paper.

5. Turn out the polenta onto a cutting board and cut into long, thin rectangles. Place on the baking sheet and sprinkle with the remaining Parmesan. Bake for 10 to 15 minutes, until the cheese has melted and the fingers are golden. Serve warm.

PER SERVING: 31 calories; 1 g protein; 2 g total fat; 1 g saturated fat; 3 g carbohydrates; 0 g fibre; 84 mg sodium

750 ml gluten-free, onion-free chicken or vegetable stock*

170 g coarse cornmeal (instant polenta)

40 g pitted black olives, finely chopped

30 g salted butter

15 g chopped flat-leaf parsley

40 g grated Parmesan

Freshly ground black pepper

* Most stocks contain onion or garlic. Choose one that is onion-free. If garlic is present, the amount is likely to be minimal and should be suitable for most people on a low-FODMAP diet. If you are extremely sensitive to garlic, omit the stock and cook the polenta in water with ½ teaspoon salt, or make your own stock by boiling chicken bones and/or suitable vegetables (including carrot and celery) in water with your choice of seasonings for about an hour, then straining out the solids.

Crispy Noodle Cakes with Chilli Sauce

MAKES 16

For presentation purposes (and to avoid making a big mess in the pan!), you can use egg rings without handles, or English muffin rings, to make these delicious cakes. Look for them in the utensil section of your supermarket. Soy sauce is always suitable for the low-FODMAP diet, as the FODMAPs have been removed. Sometimes there is wheat present, but this small amount is not a problem for people on a low-FODMAP diet. If you also follow a gluten-free diet, choose brands that are gluten-free.

1. Fill a large bowl with hot water. Add the noodles and soak for 4 to 5 minutes, until softened. Drain, then rinse under cold water and place back in the bowl. Add the coriander, ginger, five-spice powder, eggs, sesame oil, garlic-infused oil, chilli sauce, cornflour and salt and mix until well combined.

2. Heat a large heavy-bottomed frying pan over medium heat. Spray the pan and inside of the egg rings with the cooking spray (use as many rings as will fit comfortably in the pan).

3. Spoon enough noodle mixture into each ring to fill it without overflowing. Cook for 2 to 3 minutes on each side, until golden brown. Remove from the pan and run a knife around the inside of each ring to remove the noodle cakes. Set aside on a plate and cover loosely with foil to keep warm while you make the remaining cakes.

4. For the chilli sauce, combine all the ingredients in a bowl.

5. Serve the warm noodle cakes with the chilli sauce.

PER SERVING: 59 calories; 1 g protein; 3 g total fat; 1 g saturated fat; 6 g carbohydrates; 0 g fibre; 459 mg sodium

---

* Most sweet chilli sauces contain garlic. The amount present in the sauce is minimal and should be suitable for most people on a low-FODMAP diet. If you are extremely sensitive to garlic, it is best to avoid this dish, or limit intake to a very small serving. Assess your individual tolerance.

450 g dried flat rice noodles (5 mm wide), broken into 5 to 10-cm lengths

3 to 4 heaped tablespoons chopped coriander

2 teaspoons grated ginger

½ teaspoon Chinese five-spice powder

3 large eggs, lightly beaten

2 tablespoons sesame oil

2 teaspoons garlic-infused olive oil

80 ml gluten-free sweet red chilli sauce*

2 heaped tablespoons cornflour

Salt

Non-stick cooking spray

CHILLI SAUCE

125 ml gluten-free sweet red chilli sauce*

1 heaped tablespoon tomato purée

½ teaspoon gluten-free soy sauce

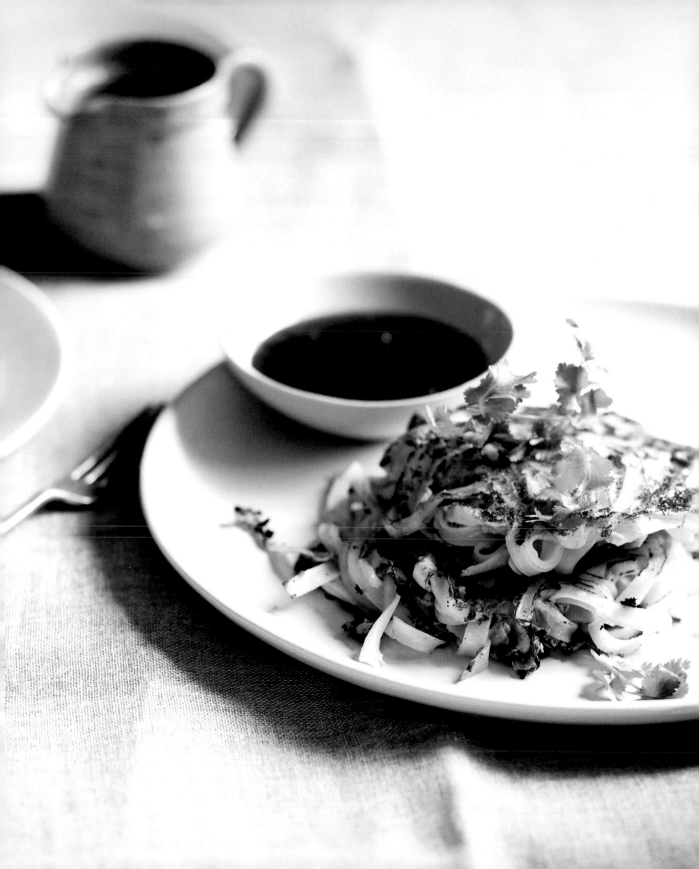

Crispy Rice Balls with Parmesan and Sweetcorn

MAKES ABOUT 30

These light finger-food treats are delicious as they are, but can also be flavoured with chopped fresh herbs such as basil, parsley, sage or lemongrass. Just use what you have on hand.

1. Pour the stock into a large saucepan and bring to a boil. Add the rice and cook until tender, 10 to 12 minutes for white rice, 45 to 50 minutes for brown. Drain and return to the pan. While the rice is still warm, stir in the Parmesan and sweetcorn. Transfer to a bowl and set aside to cool to room temperature.

2. Preheat the oven to 150°C.

3. Roll the cooled rice mixture into about 30 golf ball–size balls. Dip the balls in the beaten egg, then roll in the breadcrumbs until well coated.

4. Heat a little canola oil in a medium frying pan over medium-high heat. Working in batches of 10, add the rice balls to the pan and cook, turning regularly, until nicely browned all over. Set aside on a baking sheet and keep warm in the oven while you make the rest, adding more oil if needed. Serve warm.

PER SERVING: 45 calories; 2 g protein; 1 g total fat; 0 g saturated fat; 7 g carbohydrates; 0 g fibre; 66 mg sodium

750 ml gluten-free, onion-free chicken or vegetable stock*

150 g long-grain white or brown rice

60 g grated Parmesan

150 g tinned sweetcorn, drained

1 large egg, beaten

160 g dried gluten-free, soy-free breadcrumbs*

Canola oil, for pan-frying

---

* Most stocks contain onion or garlic. Choose one that is onion-free. If garlic is present, the amount is likely to be minimal and should be suitable for most people on a low-FODMAP diet. If you are extremely sensitive to garlic, omit the stock and cook the rice in water with ½ teaspoon salt, or make your own stock by boiling chicken bones and/or suitable vegetables (including carrot and celery) in water with your choice of seasonings for about an hour, then straining out the solids. You may make your own breadcrumbs by processing gluten-free, soy-free bread into crumbs in a food processor. Breads that include soy lecithin are suitable on the low-FODMAP diet.

Mediterranean Crustless Quiche

SERVES 6

This yummy slice is a standout meal on its own with salad, but it can also be served as an accompaniment to barbecued or grilled meat. The fresh basil gives the dish a wonderful hit of flavour, but you can use dried herbs if you prefer.

1. Preheat the oven to 170°C. Grease a 23-cm quiche dish or pie pan and line with a parchment paper circle.

2. Heat the olive oil in a non-stick frying pan over medium heat. Add the tomatoes and vinegar and cook until softened.

3. Transfer the tomatoes to a large bowl. Add the courgette, cheddar, Parmesan, eggs, basil and salt and pepper and mix to combine. Pour the quiche into the baking dish.

4. Bake for 20 to 25 minutes, until firm and lightly golden. Let stand for 5 minutes before slicing.

PER SERVING: 215 calories; 15 g protein; 15 g total fat; 7 g saturated fat; 5 g carbohydrates; 1 g fibre; 415 mg sodium

2 teaspoons olive oil

2 tomatoes, chopped

1 tablespoon balsamic vinegar

1 large courgette, thinly sliced into ribbons

120 g grated cheddar

40 g grated Parmesan

6 large eggs, lightly beaten

3 tablespoons basil leaves

Salt and freshly ground black pepper

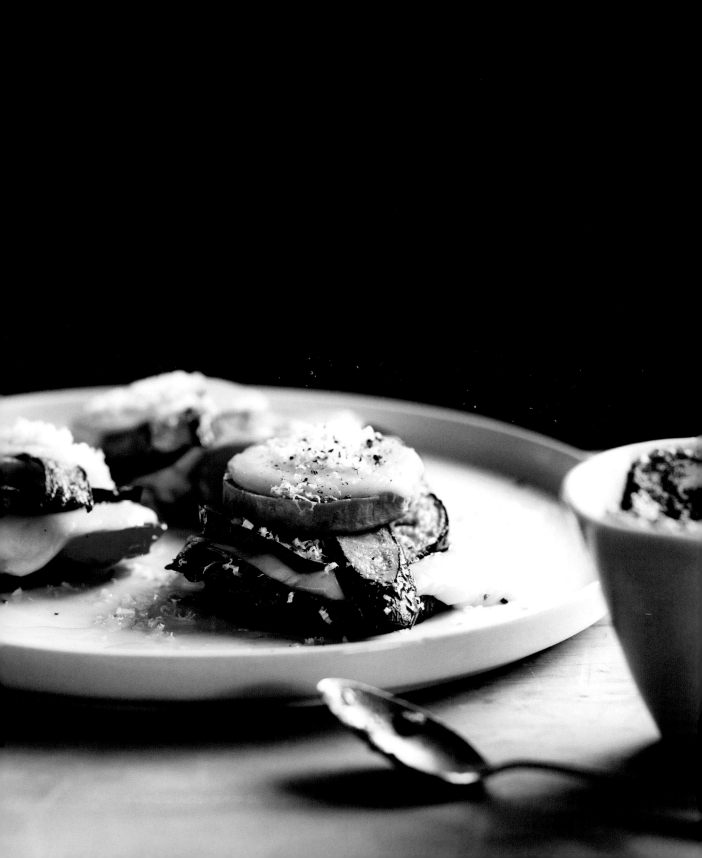

Roasted Vegetable Stacks

SERVES 4

Roasting vegetables intensifies their flavour, and they become completely irresistible when combined with homemade pesto and melted mozzarella. These are heaven as a main dish, but also delicious as a side with grilled meat, chicken or fish. If you do not eat dairy, you can leave out the Parmesan and use thinly sliced silken tofu in place of the mozzarella.

1. Preheat the oven to 170°C and line two baking sheets with parchment paper.

2. Place the aubergine and red pepper in a single layer on one sheet, and the courgette and sweet potato in a single layer on the other. Brush with a little olive oil and bake for 15 to 20 minutes, until tender.

3. On one of the baking sheets, top the aubergine slices with red pepper, courgette, and sweet potato to make stacks. Sprinkle most of the Parmesan across the stacks. Top the stacks with the mozzarella.

4. Bake for 10 to 15 minutes, until the stacks are heated through and the cheeses have melted. Season with salt and pepper and serve with a drizzle of pesto and the remaining Parmesan.

PER SERVING: 302 calories; 18 g protein; 16 g total fat; 3 g saturated fat; 24 g carbohydrates; 7 g fibre; 473 mg sodium

1 large aubergine, cut lengthwise into 5-mm slices

1 red pepper, seeded and cut into 5-cm strips

2 large courgettes, cut into 5-mm slices

1 small sweet potato, peeled (if desired) and cut into 5-mm slices

Olive oil

60 g grated Parmesan

113 g mozzarella, thinly sliced

Salt and freshly ground black pepper

35 g Basil Pesto (page 64)

Stuffed Roasted Red Peppers

SERVES 4

These have a fabulous smoky flavour and are so easy to make. To make the dish vegetarian, use crumbled gluten-free tempeh in place of the beef. To make it vegan, replace the Parmesan with an extra 30 g of pine nuts run through a food processor until crumbly.

1. Bring a large pot of water to a boil over high heat. Meanwhile, cut the tops off the red peppers and remove the stems and seeds. Using metal tongs, hold a pepper over the flame of a gas hob to char the outside evenly all over. The skin will blacken and bubble. (Alternatively, lay all the peppers on a foil-lined baking sheet and grill for 5 minutes, turning with tongs occasionally.) Place in a plastic bag and set aside to sweat. Repeat with the remaining peppers. Set aside in the bag while you make the filling.

2. Add the rice to the boiling water, decrease the heat to medium-high and cook for 10 minutes or until tender. Drain and set aside.

3. Preheat the oven to 170°C.

4. Heat the garlic-infused oil in a large frying pan over medium heat. Add the beef, paprika and thyme and cook, stirring, until the meat is nicely browned, breaking up any lumps as you go. Push the meat to the side of the pan, add the tomatoes and olive oil, and cook until the tomatoes have softened. Stir into the meat. Add the rice, vinegar, pine nuts and Parmesan. Season with the salt and pepper and stir well to combine.

5. Remove the peppers from the plastic bag and peel off the blackened skin. Small fragments of blackened skin may remain, which is fine; it will add a nice smoky flavour to the dish.

6. Spoon the meat filling evenly into the pepper shells, place them on a baking sheet, and sprinkle with a little extra Parmesan. Bake for 20 to 25 minutes, until heated through. Serve warm or cold.

PER SERVING: 672 calories; 33 g protein; 29 g total fat; 11 g saturated fat; 68 g carbohydrates; 4 g fibre; 496 mg sodium

4 red peppers

300 g white rice

1 tablespoon garlic-infused olive oil

700 g lean minced beef

1 teaspoon smoked paprika

Leaves from 8 thyme sprigs

3 large ripe tomatoes, peeled, seeded, and roughly chopped

1 teaspoon olive oil

Splash of balsamic vinegar

1 heaped tablespoon pine nuts

40 g grated Parmesan, plus more for sprinkling

Salt and freshly ground black pepper

Spring Rolls

MAKES 12

When living with food intolerances, it is often the foods we used to enjoy when eating out that we miss the most. If it's Chinese food you miss, these crisp and flavourful rolls may bridge the culinary gap.

1. Combine the garlic-infused oil, rice bran oil, ginger, five-spice powder, soy sauce, pork, carrot, bamboo shoots and cabbage in a medium bowl. Cover and refrigerate for at least 2 hours to allow the flavours to blend and the vegetables to soften.

2. Fill a large shallow dish with hot water. Place a spring roll wrapper in the water and soak for about 1 minute or until just softened. Blot on paper towels or a clean tea towel until thoroughly dry.

3. Place 2 heaped tablespoons of the filling on the bottom third of the wrapper in a line about 4 cm long. Roll the wrapper over the filling once from the bottom and fold in the sides to enclose the filling, then roll up tightly like a cigar. Arrange on a platter and cover with a moist cloth while you make the remaining rolls. Place in the refrigerator for at least 2 hours.

4. Preheat the oven to 150°C. Pour the rice bran oil into a deep-fryer or large heavy-bottomed saucepan until two-thirds full and heat over medium-high heat to 180°C; a cube of bread dropped in the oil will brown in 15 seconds, or small bubbles will appear around the handle of a wooden spoon dipped into it.

5. Working in small batches, add the spring rolls and deep-fry for 5 to 6 minutes, until crisp and golden. Remove with a slotted spoon and drain on paper towels. Keep warm in the oven while you cook the remaining spring rolls.

6. Serve hot with soy sauce, if desired.

PER SERVING (not including the extra soy sauce for dipping): 204 calories; 7 g protein; 11 g total fat; 3 g saturated fat; 20 g carbohydrates; 1 g fibre; 400 mg sodium

2 teaspoons garlic-infused olive oil

2 teaspoons rice bran oil, sunflower oil or canola oil, plus enough for deep-frying

1 teaspoon finely grated ginger

2 teaspoons Chinese five-spice powder

2 tablespoons plus 2 teaspoons gluten-free soy sauce, plus more for serving (optional)

225 g minced pork

½ carrot, finely grated

Half a 225-g tin bamboo shoots, drained well and finely chopped (70 g drained)

160 g finely shredded cabbage

Twelve 22-cm round spring roll wrappers

Rice Paper Rolls
with Dipping Sauce

MAKES ABOUT 24

These are light and fresh, not deep-fried – in fact, the rolls are not cooked at all. A simple but important key to success, as for the spring rolls, is to soak the wrappers until they are pliable but not waterlogged. And don't forget to blot them dry!

1. Fill a large bowl with very hot water. Add the noodles and soak for 4 to 5 minutes, until softened. Drain and rinse under cold water, then drain again.

2. Meanwhile, toss the chicken strips in the sweet chilli sauce. Spray a frying pan with cooking spray, add the chicken and cook over medium heat for 1 to 2 minutes, until cooked through. Set aside to cool.

3. Fill a large shallow dish with hot water. Place a spring roll wrapper in the water and soak for about 1 minute or until just softened. Blot dry on paper towels or a clean tea towel.

4. Place a small handful of noodles on the bottom third of the wrapper and top with a little shredded lettuce and two or three pieces of carrot and chicken in a line about 4 cm long. Top with a sprinkling of coriander. Roll the wrapper over the filling once from the bottom and fold in the sides to enclose the filling, then roll up tightly like a cigar. Arrange on a platter and cover with a moist cloth while you make the remaining rolls. Cover with cling film and refrigerate if not serving immediately.

5. Serve the rolls with a small bowl of sweet chilli sauce for dipping.

PER SERVING (1/24 recipe, with chilli sauce for dipping): 75 calories; 3 g protein; 1 g total fat; 0 g saturated fat; 14 g carbohydrates; 0 g fibre; 71 mg sodium

100 g gluten-free rice vermicelli, broken into 10-cm lengths

200 g boneless, skinless chicken thighs, thinly sliced

60 ml gluten-free sweet red chilli sauce,* plus more for serving

Non-stick cooking spray

Twenty-four 22-cm round rice paper wrappers

1 small head butter lettuce (Boston or Bibb), leaves shredded

1 small carrot, thinly sliced into 3-cm strips

Handful of coriander leaves

---

* Most sweet chilli sauces contain garlic. The amount present in the sauce is minimal and should be suitable for most people on a low-FODMAP diet. If you are extremely sensitive to garlic, it is best to avoid this dish, or limit intake to a very small serving. Assess your individual tolerance.

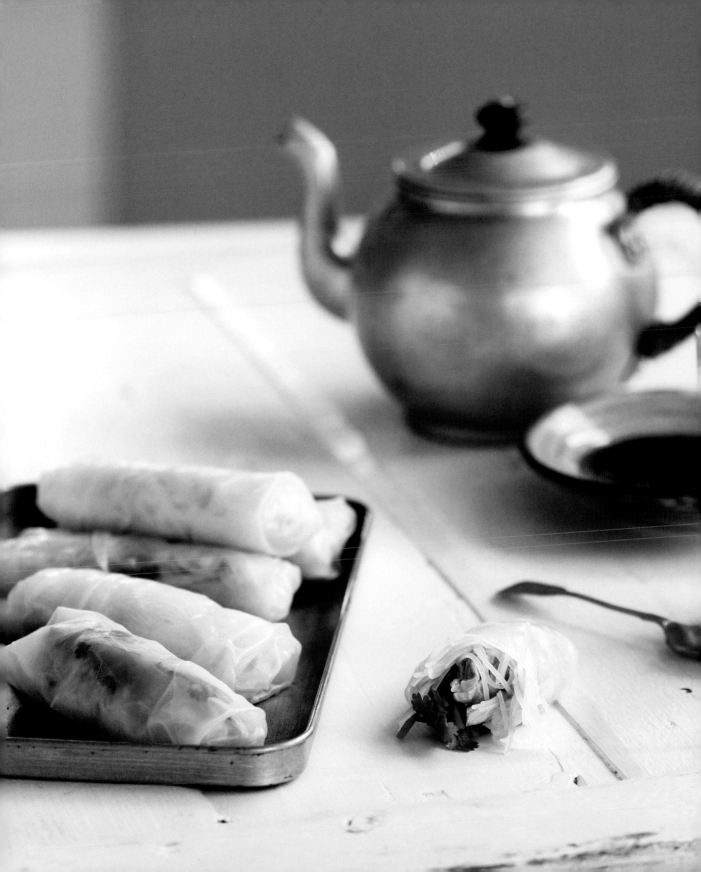

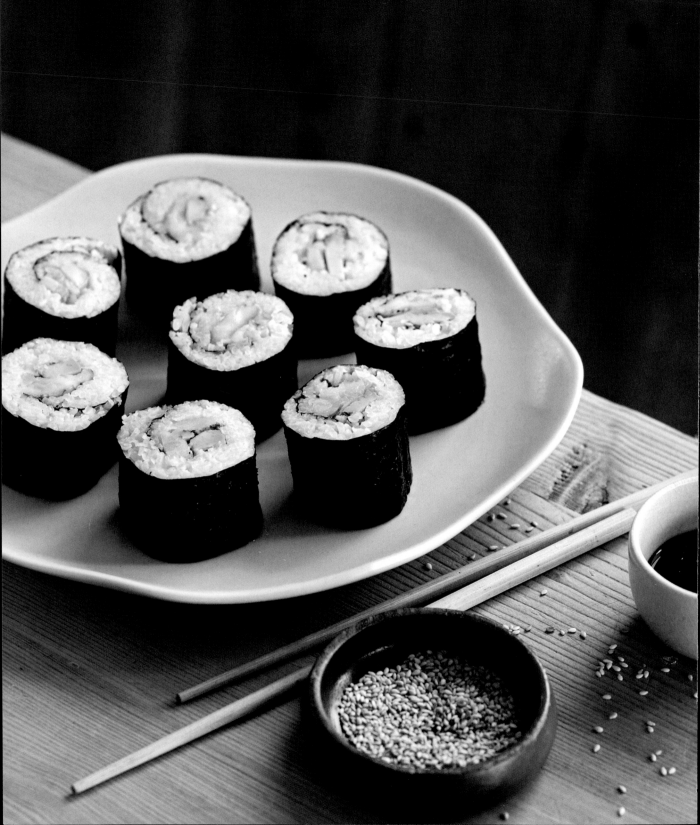

Sushi

MAKES 12

These are so easy to make, and the fillings can be as varied as your imagination (and pantry) will allow. I have given a few suggestions below to get you started.

1. Place the rice and 1 litre water in large saucepan. Bring to a boil, reduce the heat to medium-low, cover, and cook for 8 minutes. Remove from the heat and let stand, still covered, for 10 minutes.

2. Combine the vinegar, sugar and salt in a small bowl and stir until the sugar has dissolved.

3. Transfer the rice to a large bowl, add the vinegar mixture and gently stir to make the rice grains slightly sticky but still separated. Cover with a damp tea towel and keep warm. Do not refrigerate.

4. Place a sheet of nori on a sushi mat or piece of parchment paper, shiny-side down, with the longer edge closest to you. Spread one-sixth of the cooked rice over the closer two-thirds of the nori sheet in a 3 to 5 mm-thick layer. Place your chosen filling across the centre of the rice layer. Pick up the nori edge closer to you and roll it over the filling, using the sushi mat or parchment paper to help you. Keep rolling it firmly until you reach the end of the sheet. Wet the end with a little water and press gently to seal. Set aside, seam-side down, and repeat with the remaining nori, rice and fillings.

5. Refrigerate for 1 hour, covered with cling film. Use a sharp knife to cut the rolls in half or into smaller pieces. Serve with wasabi paste, toasted sesame seeds and soy sauce.

SUSHI PER SERVING:

Prawn and avocado (not including the wasabi or soy sauce): 199 calories; 5 g protein; 3 g total fat; 0 g saturated fat; 36 g carbohydrates; 2 g fibre; 114 mg sodium

Vegetarian (not including the wasabi or soy sauce): 255 calories; 6 g protein; 8 g total fat; 1 g saturated fat; 37 g carbohydrates; 3 g fibre; 190 mg sodium

Smoked salmon (not including the wasabi, soy sauce or sesame seeds): 241 calories; 7 g protein; 7 g total fat; 1 g saturated fat; 36 g carbohydrates; 2 g fibre; 307 mg sodium

500 g short-grain (sushi) rice

80 ml seasoned rice vinegar

1 heaped tablespoon caster sugar

½ teaspoon salt

6 nori sheets

Gluten-free wasabi paste, toasted sesame seeds and gluten-free soy sauce, for serving

FILLINGS SUGGESTIONS

Prawn and avocado: 12 peeled cooked prawns (halved lengthwise), avocado slices and toasted sesame seeds

Vegetarian: avocado slices, baked or fried tofu strips, carrot matchsticks, shredded lettuce, cucumber strips, gluten-free mayonnaise and toasted sesame seeds

Smoked salmon: smoked salmon strips or flaked tinned tuna, avocado slices (optional), cucumber strips and gluten-free mayonnaise

Dim Sims
(Pork and Prawn Dumplings)

MAKES 24

These Chinese-inspired dumplings may seem fussy to make, but they are well worth it. You can make up batches in advance and reheat them in a 150°C oven to accompany any Asian-inspired dish, such as Rice Paper Rolls with Dipping Sauce (page 42). Kitchen string is available from kitchen and homeware stores.

1. Preheat the oven to 150°C.
2. Combine the pork, prawns, bamboo shoots and cabbage in a medium bowl. Combine the egg, soy sauce, sesame oil, garlic-infused oil, ginger and cornflour in a small bowl and whisk until smooth. Pour the sauce over the pork mixture and mix until well combined.
3. Fill a large shallow dish with hot water. Place a spring roll wrapper in the water and soak for about 1 minute or until just softened. Blot dry on paper towels or a clean tea towel.
4. Place 2 tablespoons of the pork mixture in the centre of the wrapper. Gather the wrapper up in the middle and tie in a bow with kitchen string. Arrange on a platter and cover with a moist cloth while you make the remaining dumplings.
5. Pour the canola oil into a deep-fryer or large heavy-bottomed saucepan until two-thirds full and heat over medium-high heat to 180°C; a cube of bread dropped in the oil will brown in 15 seconds, or small bubbles will appear around the handle of a wooden spoon dipped into it. Add a small batch of dumplings and deep-fry for 5 minutes or until crisp and golden. Remove with a slotted spoon and drain on paper towel. Untie the string and keep the dumplings warm in the oven while you cook the rest.
6. Serve hot with soy sauce.

450 g minced pork

150 g raw prawns, peeled and deveined, finely chopped

One 225-g tin bamboo shoots, drained and finely chopped (about 160 g)

80 g finely chopped cabbage

1 large egg, lightly beaten

2 tablespoons plus 2 teaspoons gluten-free soy sauce, plus more for serving

2 teaspoons sesame oil

2 teaspoons garlic-infused olive oil

1½ teaspoons finely grated ginger

1 heaped tablespoon cornflour

Twenty-four 16-cm round spring roll wrappers

Canola, soybean, safflower, rice bran or sunflower oil, for deep-frying

PER SERVING (not including the extra soy sauce for dipping): 165 calories; 7 g protein; 10 g total fat; 2 g saturated fat; 12 g carbohydrates; 1 g fibre; 231 mg sodium

Salmon and Prawn Skewers

SERVES 4

This naturally low-FODMAP summer dish is sure to be a hit with your friends. Make sure you get the very freshest salmon and prawns possible.

1. Place the salmon and prawns in a glass or ceramic bowl. Combine the olive oil, lime juice and zest, cayenne pepper, salt and pepper in a small bowl. Pour over the salmon and prawns and toss well to combine. Cover and refrigerate for 2 to 3 hours to marinate.

2. If using wooden skewers, soak them in water for about 10 minutes to prevent scorching (you will need eight skewers for this recipe).

3. Thread alternate pieces of salmon and prawns onto the skewers.

4. Pan-fry or grill the skewers until the seafood is just cooked (no longer translucent). Serve with a fresh green salad.

PER SERVING (not including the green salad): 382 calories; 38 g protein; 24 g total fat; 4 g saturated fat; 1 g carbohydrates; 0 g fibre; 296 mg sodium

600 g boneless, skinless Atlantic salmon steaks or fillet, cut into 2-cm cubes

24 raw large prawns, peeled and deveined, tails intact

60 ml olive oil

2 tablespoons plus 2 teaspoons fresh lime juice

2 to 3 teaspoons finely grated lime zest

¼ teaspoon cayenne pepper

½ teaspoon salt

Freshly ground black pepper

Green salad, for serving

Sesame Prawns with Coriander Salad

SERVES 4

It isn't difficult to master a light, crispy batter that is wheat-free. An electric deep-fryer is helpful because you can set the thermometer to the exact temperature required, but if you don't have one, a good heavy-bottomed saucepan will do the job.

1. Combine the egg, sesame seeds, 150 g of the cornflour, and 170 ml water in a medium bowl. Mix until well combined with no lumps. Refrigerate for 30 minutes.

2. To make the salad, combine the lettuce, cucumber, celery, pepper, coriander and mint in a large bowl. Whisk together the lemon juice, vinegar, sugar and chilli (if using) in a small bowl. Refrigerate the salad and dressing separately until just before serving.

3. Half-fill a deep-fryer or large heavy-bottomed saucepan with oil and heat over medium-high heat to 180°C; a cube of bread dropped in the oil will brown in 15 seconds, or small bubbles will appear around the handle of a wooden spoon dipped into it.

4. Remove the batter from the fridge and stir. Toss the prawns in the remaining cornflour and shake off any excess. Dip the prawns in the batter and drop immediately into the heated oil in small batches. Cook for 3 to 4 minutes, until the batter is crispy. Remove the prawns with a slotted spoon and drain on paper towels while you fry the rest.

5. As the last batch of prawns cooks, pour the dressing over the salad and gently toss to coat. Serve the prawns immediately with the salad.

PER SERVING: 366 calories; 10 g protein; 16 g total fat; 2 g saturated fat; 45 g carbohydrates; 3 g fibre; 69 mg sodium

1 large egg

35 g sesame seeds, toasted

185 g cornflour

CORIANDER SALAD

150 g roughly chopped lettuce leaves

½ cucumber, diced

2 celery stalks, thinly sliced

½ green pepper, seeded and diced

Handful of coriander leaves

Small handful of mint leaves

2 tablespoons plus 2 teaspoons fresh lemon juice

1 tablespoon plus 1 teaspoon seasoned rice vinegar

2 teaspoons sugar

½ small chilli, seeded and finely chopped (optional)

Canola, soybean, safflower, rice bran or sunflower oil, for deep-frying

16 raw large prawns, peeled and deveined, tails intact

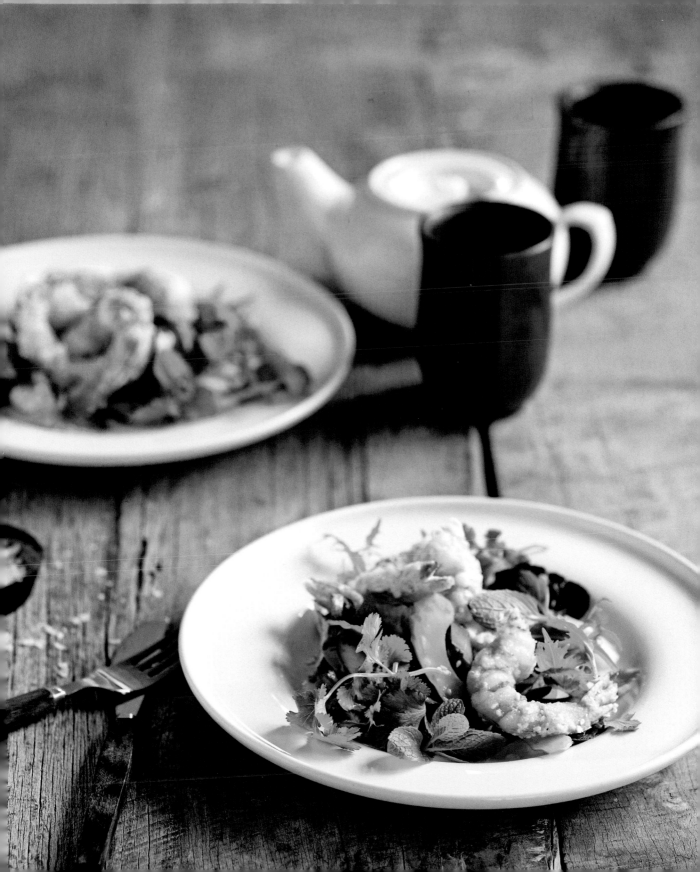

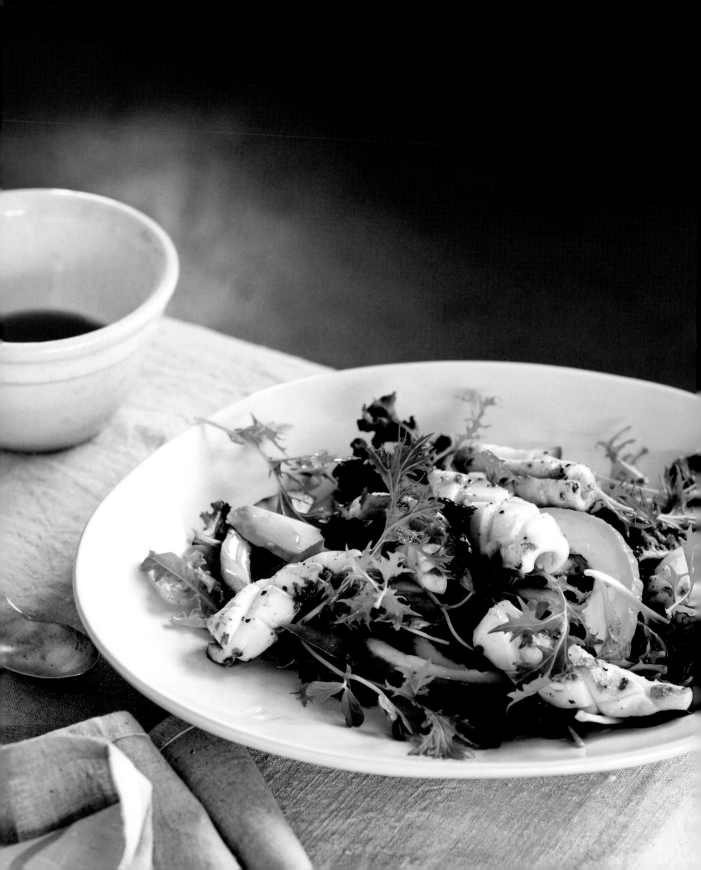

Salt-and-Pepper Calamari with Green Salad

SERVES 4

This simple dish, when found on Chinese restaurant menus, is normally a safe bet for those following a low-FODMAP diet. But if you want to try cooking it at home, it isn't hard to do. Just grab a few fresh ingredients and follow the recipe below.

1. Using a sharp knife, score the squid pieces in a 1-cm criss-cross pattern. Take care not to cut all the way through – just about three quarters of the way. This ensures the squid will curl when cooked.

2. Combine the garlic-infused oil, olive oil, salt and pepper in a large bowl. Add the squid pieces and toss to coat. Cover and refrigerate for 3 to 4 hours.

3. Shortly before you're ready to eat, prepare the salad. Combine the lettuce, cucumber, avocado (if using), celery, green pepper and pea shoots in a large bowl.

4. To make the dressing, combine all the ingredients in a small screw-top jar and shake until well mixed.

5. Preheat a grill to high (or place a ridged grill pan or cast-iron frying pan over high heat). Add the squid and cook for 3 to 4 minutes, until curled and lightly golden.

6. Shake the dressing again if it has separated, drizzle over the salad, and toss gently to coat. Divide among individual plates and arrange the squid on top. Serve immediately.

PER SERVING: 475 calories; 29 g protein; 34 g total fat; 6 g saturated fat; 15 g carbohydrates; 4 g fibre; 394 mg sodium

8 medium squid bodies, well cleaned and cut into quarters

1 tablespoon garlic-infused olive oil

2 tablespoons olive oil

½ teaspoon salt

Freshly ground black pepper

GREEN SALAD

150 g roughly chopped lettuce leaves

½ cucumber, thinly sliced

1 avocado, pitted, peeled and sliced (optional)

2 celery stalks, thinly sliced

½ green pepper, seeded and sliced

50 g pea shoots or bean sprouts

DRESSING

60 ml olive oil

2 tablespoons fresh lemon juice

1 tablespoon garlic-infused olive oil

½ teaspoon brown sugar

Salt

San Choy Bow
(Asian Pork Lettuce Wraps)

SERVES 6

This dish is all about freshness, so make sure you use vibrant green lettuce leaves to hold the filling. Choose medium leaves that are similar in size.

1. Heat a wok over medium-high heat. Pour in the sesame oil and garlic-infused oil and heat until almost smoking. Add the ginger and stir-fry until lightly browned. Add the pork and stir-fry over high heat for 3 to 4 minutes, until well browned, breaking up any lumps as you go.

2. Add the bamboo shoots, water chestnuts, coriander, lemon juice, sweet chilli sauce and fish sauce and stir-fry for 2 minutes more.

3. Arrange the lettuce on a platter or individual plates, convex side down (like cups). Use a slotted spoon to spoon the pork filling into the lettuce cups and serve immediately.

PER SERVING: 301 calories; 14 g protein; 23 g total fat; 7 g saturated fat; 9 g carbohydrates; 3 g fibre; 164 mg sodium

---

* Most sweet chilli sauces contain garlic. The amount present in the sauce is minimal and should be suitable for most people on a low-FODMAP diet. If you are extremely sensitive to garlic, omit the sweet chilli sauce from this recipe.

2 tablespoons sesame oil

1 tablespoon garlic-infused olive oil

2 teaspoons finely grated ginger

450 g minced pork

One 225-g tin bamboo shoots, drained and finely chopped

One 225-g can water chestnuts, drained and finely chopped

1 heaped tablespoon chopped coriander

2 tablespoons plus 2 teaspoons fresh lemon juice

2 tablespoons gluten-free sweet red chilli sauce*

1 teaspoon fish sauce, or ¾ teaspoon soy sauce and a splash of lime juice

6 iceberg lettuce leaves, rinsed and dried

Oysters, Three Ways

MAKES 12

When it comes to oysters, fresh is always best. Get them from a reputable fishmonger on the day you plan to eat them. When buying them in the shell, the oysters should look and smell clean and be sitting firmly within the shell. Each of the topping options makes enough for twelve oysters, so take your pick. Oysters Kilpatrick have a delicate mix of flavours – the Worcestershire sauce offers sweetness, the bacon a salty smokiness. I'm sure you'll find it hard to stop at just one!

1. Line a baking sheet with foil and place the oysters in their shells on the sheet. Preheat the grill to high.

2. For cheese-crusted oysters, combine the breadcrumbs, Parmesan and parsley in a small bowl. Place a slice of Camembert on each oyster. Sprinkle the breadcrumb mixture over the top.

3. For oysters Kilpatrick, cook the bacon until crisp. Drain on a paper towel. Place 1 teaspoon bacon and 1 teaspoon Worcestershire sauce on each oyster.

4. For tomato and chilli oysters, heat the oil in a small frying pan over medium heat, add the chilli pepper, and cook until softened. Stir in the tomato passata. Spoon the sauce evenly over the oysters.

5. Place the oysters under the grill and cook for a few minutes until warmed through. Serve immediately, but be careful, because the shells will be hot!

PER SERVING:

Cheese-Crusted: 38 calories; 3 g protein; 2 g total fat; 1 g saturated fat; 1 g carbohydrates; 0 g fibre; 104 mg sodium

Kilpatrick: 55 calories; 4 g protein; 5 g total fat; 1 g saturated fat; 2 g carbohydrates; 0 g fibre; 253 mg sodium

Tomato and chilli:19 calories; 1 g protein; 1 g total fat; 0 g saturated fat; 2 g carbohydrates; 0 g fibre; 66 mg sodium

12 freshly shucked oysters, fully detached from and replaced on their shell

CHEESE-CRUSTED

2 heaped tablespoons dried gluten-free, soy-free breadcrumbs*

1 heaped tablespoon grated Parmesan

1 teaspoon finely chopped flat-leaf parsley

100 g Camembert, cut into 12 thin slices

OYSTERS KILPATRICK

3 to 5 lean bacon slices (100 g), finely chopped

60 ml gluten-free Worcestershire sauce*

TOMATO AND CHILLI

2 teaspoons garlic-infused olive oil

½ small red chilli pepper, finely chopped

125 ml tomato passata

---

* You may make your own breadcrumbs by processing gluten-free, soy-free bread into crumbs in a food processor. Breads that include soy lecithin are suitable. Most Worcestershire sauces contain a minimal amount of garlic. In small amounts it should be suitable, but if you are extremely sensitive to garlic, opt for the cheese-crusted or tomato and chilli oysters.

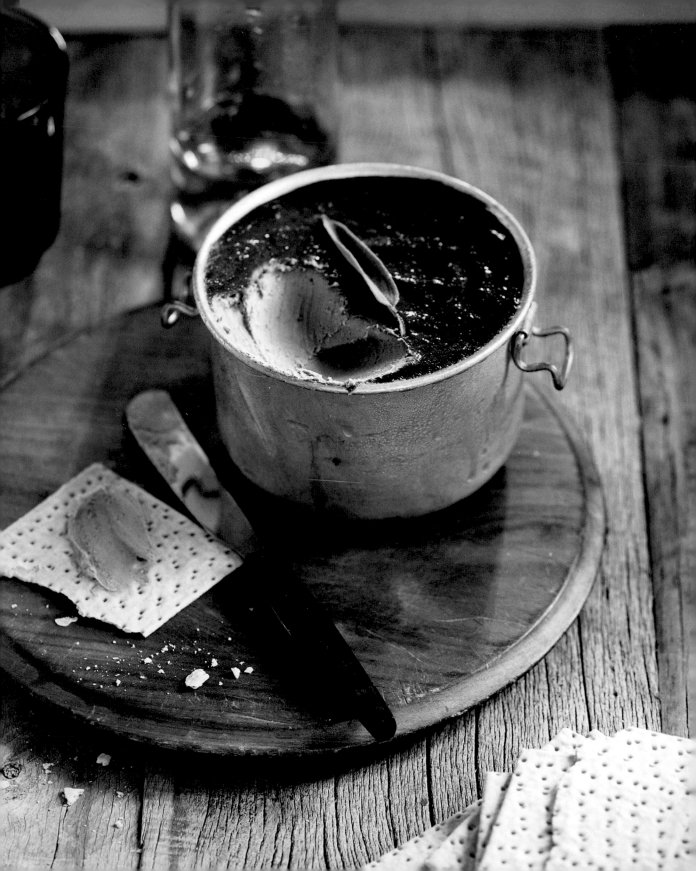

Chicken Liver Pâté with Pepper and Sage

SERVES 12

Most pâtés contain onion, which puts them off the menu for low-FODMAP eaters. This onion-free recipe is inexpensive, easy to make and tastes amazing – I think you will be very pleased with the result.

1. Combine the 115 g butter, garlic-infused oil and olive oil in a medium saucepan over medium heat. Add the sage and cook for 2 to 3 minutes, stirring regularly. Add the chicken livers and cook until just browned. Remove from the heat and stir in the pepper and cream. Purée with an immersion blender or in a food processor until smooth. Add the melted butter and blend until combined.

2. Pour into six 125-m ramekins or one 700-ml mould and garnish with the sage leaves. Cover and refrigerate for 3 hours or until set.

3. Serve with crackers.

PER SERVING (not including the crackers): 185 calories; 8 g protein; 16 g total fat; 9 g saturated fat; 2 g carbohydrates; 0 g fibre; 144 mg sodium

115 g unsalted butter, plus 45 g melted butter

1 tablespoon garlic-infused olive oil

1 tablespoon olive oil

1 teaspoon finely chopped sage, plus more leaves for garnish

500 g chicken livers, rinsed and trimmed (about 10 livers)

1 heaped tablespoon freshly ground black pepper

125 ml single cream

Gluten-free crackers, for serving

Crêpes with Cheese Sauce

SERVES 4

I remember visiting crêperies with my family as a young girl and really enjoying the meals we ate. Because you can change the filling flavours to suit individual preferences, it's the perfect family dish.

1. To make the crêpes, sift the rice flour, cornflour, soy flour and baking soda three times into a large bowl (or whisk in the bowl until well combined). Make a well in the middle, add the eggs and milk and blend to form a smooth batter. Stir in the melted butter. Cover with cling film and set aside for 20 minutes.

2. Heat a heavy-bottomed frying pan or crêpe pan over medium heat and spray well with cooking spray. Pour about 60 ml batter into the warmed pan and tilt to coat the bottom thinly. Cook until bubbles start to appear, then carefully turn the crêpe over and briefly cook the other side. Transfer to a platter and cover loosely with foil to keep warm while you repeat with the remaining batter (to make 8 crêpes in total) and make the cheese sauce.

3. To make the cheese sauce, blend 60 ml of the milk with the cornflour to make a paste. Add the remaining milk, whisking well to avoid any lumps. Pour the mixture into a small saucepan and stir over medium heat until thickened. (Don't let it boil.) Add the cheddar and stir until melted. Season to taste with salt and pepper. Keep warm while you prepare the filling of your choice.

4. To make the ham and spinach filling, heat the olive oil in a large frying pan over medium heat. Add the spinach and stir to coat in the oil. Cover the pan and cook for about 1 minute, then uncover, stir, cover again and continue to cook until just wilted, about 1 minute more. Divide the spinach evenly between the crêpes and top with the sliced ham.

CRÊPES

100 g superfine white rice flour

75 g cornflour

30 g soy flour

¾ teaspoon baking soda

2 large eggs, lightly beaten

375 ml semi-skimmed milk, lactose-free milk or suitable plant-based milk

45 g salted butter, melted

Non-stick cooking spray

CHEESE SAUCE

500 ml semi-skimmed milk, lactose-free milk or suitable plant-based milk

2 heaped tablespoons cornflour

240 g grated reduced-fat cheddar

Salt and freshly ground black pepper

HAM AND SPINACH FILLING

Olive oil, for pan-frying

225 g baby spinach leaves, rinsed and dried

225 g thinly sliced gluten-free smoked ham

5. To make the tempeh and rice filling, heat the garlic-infused oil in a large frying pan over medium-high heat. Add the crumbled tempeh, smoked paprika and thyme and sauté until browned and crisp, about 7 minutes. Add the rice and continue to sauté until the rice is warmed through. Remove from the heat and stir in the tomatoes, olive oil, balsamic vinegar and salt and pepper. Divide the filling evenly between the crêpes and top each with a sprinkle of pine nuts.

6. Top the crêpes with a drizzle of the cheese sauce and your choice of filling and fold to enclose. Serve with the remaining cheese sauce and a final grinding of pepper.

CRÊPES WITH CHEESE SAUCE PER SERVING:
Ham and Spinach Filling: 670 calories; 41 g protein; 30 g total fat; 18 g saturated fat; 55 g carbohydrates; 4 g fibre; 1919 mg sodium

Tempeh and Rice Filling: 676 calories; 36 g protein; 31 g total fat; 12 g saturated fat; 65 g carbohydrates; 3 g fibre; 651 mg sodium

TEMPEH AND RICE FILLING

½ tablespoon garlic-infused olive oil

360 g crumbled gluten-free tempeh

½ teaspoon smoked paprika

Leaves from 4 thyme sprigs

140 g cooked white rice

2 medium ripe tomatoes, peeled, seeded and roughly chopped

½ teaspoon olive oil

Splash of balsamic vinegar

Salt and freshly ground black pepper to taste

40 g pine nuts

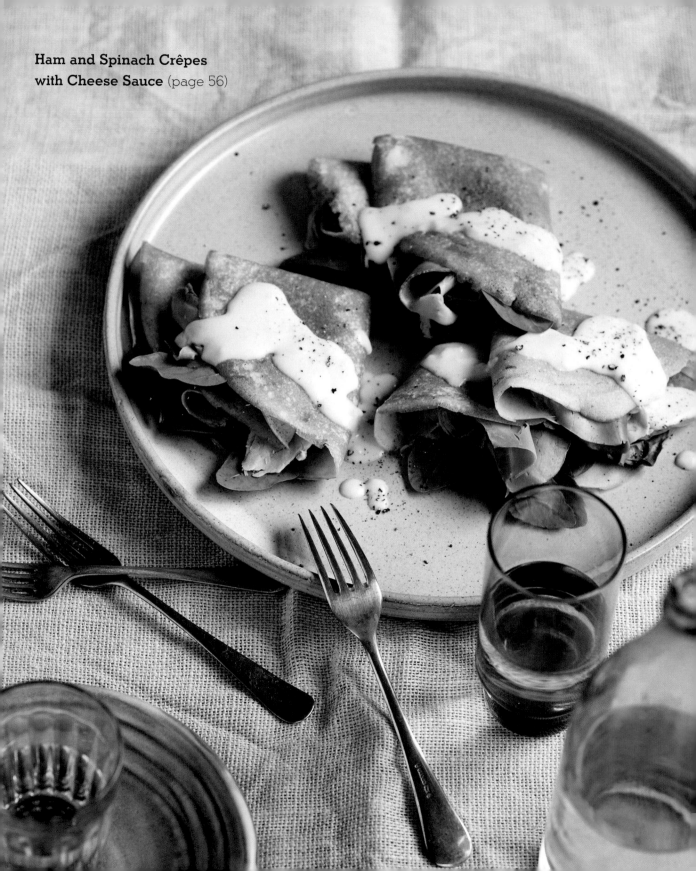

Ham and Spinach Crêpes
with Cheese Sauce (page 56)

Spinach, Squash and Sage Polenta Squares

SERVES 4

I love the fact that polenta can be a base for so many flavour combinations. This time I'm enjoying it with a mix of sage, squash and spinach, and I'm sure you will too. It's delicious served with Green Salad (see page 51).

1. Preheat the oven to 180°C.

2. Place the squash pieces on a baking sheet and drizzle with the oil. Bake for 30 to 40 minutes, until cooked through and golden, turning occasionally. Cover with foil and set aside.

3. Bring the stock to a boil in a medium saucepan over high heat. Add the cornmeal, reduce the heat to medium-low, and cook, stirring constantly, for 2 to 3 minutes. By this stage the polenta should be very thick. Remove from the heat. Add 2 table-spoons of oil and the sage and spinach, and stir until the spinach has wilted. Season to taste with salt and pepper.

4. Line an 20-cm square baking dish with parchment paper and arrange the squash pieces over the bottom. Pour the polenta over the top and smooth the surface. Allow to cool slightly, cover with cling film, and refrigerate for 2 to 3 hours, until firm.

5. Turn out the polenta onto a cutting board and cut into pieces. Enjoy it cold, or warm it on foil under the grill for 3 to 5 minutes. It's also delicious heated on the stove in a ridged griddle pan or cast-iron frying pan.

6. Serve with a green salad.

PER SERVING (not including the green salad): 191 calories; 4 g protein; 5 g total fat; 1 g saturated fat; 37 g carbohydrates; 4 g fibre; 470 mg sodium

---

* Most stocks contain onion or garlic. Choose one that is onion-free. If garlic is present, the amount is likely to be minimal and should be suitable for most people on a low-FODMAP diet. If you are extremely sensitive to garlic, replace the stock with water, or make your own stock by boiling suitable vegetables (including carrot and celery) in water with your choice of seasonings for about an hour, then straining out the solids.

400 g kabocha or other suitable winter squash, peeled, seeded and cut into 2-cm cubes

Garlic-infused olive oil

750 ml gluten-free, onion-free vegetable stock*

170 g coarse cornmeal (instant polenta)

2 tablespoons roughly chopped sage leaves

60 g baby spinach leaves, rinsed and dried

Salt and freshly ground black pepper

Green salad, for serving

Pesto Mini Pizzas

SERVES 6

Bread mix works really well for pizza crusts, whether miniature, as in this recipe, or full size (page 118). There are many different gluten-free bread mixes available these days – look for one with low-FODMAP ingredients (soy lecithin is suitable) in the baking section of the supermarket or in health food shops. I've suggested two topping options, one of which is vegetarian (or vegan, if you leave out the cheese in the pesto).

1. Preheat the oven to 120°C. Line one or two large baking sheets with parchment paper.

2. Prepare the bread mix following the directions on the package. Spoon one-sixth of the bread mix onto the parchment paper and spread with the back of a large metal spoon into a 15-cm circle. Dip the spoon in water if necessary to help with the spreading. Repeat with the remaining mix. Bake for 15 minutes or until lightly browned. Remove from the oven and increase the temperature to 180°C.

3. Meanwhile, for chicken and bacon pizzas, heat the oil in a heavy-bottomed frying pan over medium heat. Add the chicken and bacon and cook, stirring, until the bacon is crispy and the chicken is golden brown. Remove with a slotted spoon and drain on paper towels.

4. For the tempeh and red pepper pizzas, heat the oil in a heavy-bottomed frying pan over medium heat. Add the tempeh and cook, stirring, until crispy. Remove with a slotted spoon and drain on paper towels.

5. Spread 1 teaspoon pesto over each pizza crust. Top with the bacon and chicken and then the mozzarella, or with the tempeh and roasted peppers. Bake for 15 minutes or until the cheese has melted. For a crisper crust, bake the pizzas directly on the oven rack.

300 g gluten-free, soy-free bread mix

2 tablespoons Basil Pesto (page 64)

CHICKEN AND BACON

2 teaspoons garlic-infused olive oil

450 g boneless, skinless chicken breasts, thinly sliced

225 g lean bacon slices, chopped

6 mozzarella bocconcini, sliced

TEMPEH AND RED PEPPER

2 teaspoons garlic-infused olive oil

450 g gluten-free tempeh, crumbled and steamed

170 g roasted red peppers, sliced

PER SERVING:

Chicken and Bacon:
514 calories; 38 g protein; 27 g total fat; 8 g saturated fat; 26 g carbohydrates; 3 g fibre; 1070 mg sodium

Tempeh and Red Pepper:
323 calories; 21 g protein; 10 g total fat; 2 g saturated fat; 37 g carbohydrates; 9 g fibre; 378 mg sodium

Vegetable-Tofu Skewers

SERVES 4

Although tofu is made from soy, and soy is a legume that contains FODMAPs, I'm happy to say that tofu – because of its processing – is low in FODMAPs. So enjoy these skewers with gusto!

1. Combine the soy sauce, sesame oil and ginger in a small bowl. Place the tofu in a large container with a lid. Pour the marinade over the top and toss gently to coat. Cover and refrigerate for 2 to 3 hours, shaking occasionally to evenly coat the tofu with the marinade.

2. Bring a large pot of water to a boil. Add the sweet potato and cook over medium-high heat for about 5 minutes, until just tender. Drain and set aside.

3. If using wooden skewers, soak them in water for about 10 minutes to prevent scorching (you will need eight skewers). If grillling, preheat the grill; if griddling, preheat the pan to medium.

4. Thread the vegetable and tofu pieces onto the skewers in an alternating pattern.

5. Griddle or pan-fry the skewers over medium heat, or broil, turning regularly and brushing with a little olive oil if necessary to prevent them from sticking.

6. Serve hot, drizzled with the sweet chilli sauce.

PER SERVING (including the optional olive oil): 462 calories; 14 g protein; 19 g total fat; 3 g saturated fat; 63 g carbohydrates; 10 g fibre; 1151 mg sodium

---

* Most chilli sauces contain garlic. The amount present in the sauce is likely to be minimal and should be suitable for most people on a low-FODMAP diet. If you are extremely sensitive to garlic, it is best to avoid the sauce, or limit intake to a very small serving. Assess your individual tolerance.

125 ml gluten-free soy sauce

2 tablespoons sesame oil

1 teaspoon grated ginger

200 g firm tofu, pressed and cut into 1.5-cm cubes

500 g sweet potatoes, cut into 2-cm cubes

1 large aubergine, cut into 1.5-cm cubes

1 large courgette, halved lengthwise and cut into 1-cm slices

2 green or red peppers, seeded and cut into 2-cm squares

Olive oil (optional)

125 ml gluten-free sweet red chilli sauce*

Chicken Drumsticks with Lemon and Coriander

SERVES 4

If you have children, encourage them to join you in the kitchen to make this really easy dinner. Quick to prepare and packed full of flavour, this family favourite is delicious warm or cold. Try it with a green salad or cooked rice.

60 ml gluten-free soy sauce

2 tablespoons plus 2 teaspoons light brown sugar

2 teaspoons garlic-infused olive oil

2 teaspoons olive oil

2 tablespoons plus 2 teaspoons fresh lemon juice

2 tablespoons plus 2 teaspoons sesame oil

8 chicken drumsticks

2 heaped tablespoons chopped coriander

1. To make the marinade, combine the soy sauce, brown sugar, garlic-infused oil, olive oil, lemon juice and sesame oil in a large baking dish and stir until the sugar has dissolved.

2. Add the chicken to the marinade and turn each drumstick to make sure they are all well coated. Cover the dish and refrigerate for a few hours or overnight.

3. Preheat the oven to 180°C, or a grill to medium-high. Bake or grill the drumsticks, turning occasionally, for 15 to 20 minutes, until the juices run clear when the drumsticks are pierced in the thickest part with a toothpick. Sprinkle with the coriander just before serving.

PER SERVING: 233 calories; 26 g protein; 11 g total fat; 2 g saturated fat; 5 g carbohydrates; 0 g fibre; 566 mg sodium

Beef Kofta with Tahini Sauce

SERVES 4–6

Kofta are meatballs or croquettes generally made with spiced minced beef or lamb. In this version, they're made on skewers, though this is optional. The small amount of yogurt used in the sauce does not contain a large amount of lactose, making it suitable for people with lactose intolerance.

1. If using wooden skewers, soak them in water for 10 minutes to prevent scorching (you will need 12 skewers).If grilling, preheat the grill.

2. Meanwhile, make the tahini sauce by whisking all the ingredients together in a small bowl. Set aside to allow the flavours to meld.

3. Combine the beef, eggs, breadcrumbs, parsley, cinnamon, cumin, cayenne pepper, turmeric and allspice in a large bowl and mix with your hands until well combined. Shape about 60 g of the beef mixture around each skewer.

4. Grill, griddle or pan-fry the kofta until browned all over and cooked to your preferred doneness.

5. Serve with the tahini sauce and your choice of salad or vegetables.

PER SERVING (⅙ recipe; not including the salad): 347 calories; 24 g protein; 23 g total fat; 8 g saturated fat; 8 g carbohydrates; 2 g fibre; 122 mg sodium

---

* You may make your own breadcrumbs by processing gluten-free, soy-free bread into crumbs in a food processor. Breads that include soy lecithin are suitable on the low-FODMAP diet.

TAHINI SAUCE

140 g gluten-free low-fat plain yogurt

2 teaspoons fresh lemon juice

2 tablespoons plus 2 teaspoons tahini

1 teaspoon garlic-infused olive oil

600 g lean minced beef

2 large eggs, lightly beaten

40 g dried gluten-free, soy-free breadcrumbs*

15 g finely chopped flat-leaf parsley

1 teaspoon ground cinnamon

2 tablespoons ground cumin

½ teaspoon cayenne pepper, or to taste

1 heaped tablespoon ground turmeric

1½ teaspoons ground allspice

Green salad or vegetables, for serving

DIPS & SAUCES

EACH RECIPE MAKES 200 G

These dips and sauces are absolute staples in my fridge. They can be enjoyed simply with gluten-free bread, crackers or fresh vegetables; spooned over grilled meats or vegetables; spread over a pizza crust; or stirred into gluten-free pasta. The fresh, intense flavours will lift whatever you pair them with.

Salsa Verde

2 handfuls of flat-leaf parsley, rinsed and dried
3 anchovy fillets in oil, drained (optional)
2 teaspoons capers, rinsed and drained
1 tablespoon garlic-infused olive oil
2 tablespoons olive oil
2 tablespoons fresh lemon juice, or to taste
Salt and freshly ground black pepper

Combine the parsley, anchovy fillets (if using) and capers in a food processor or blender and process until well combined. Gradually add the garlic-infused oil and olive oil until well blended. Add the lemon juice and salt and pepper to taste. Spoon into a bowl or jar, cover and store in the fridge for up to 5 days.

PER SERVING (1 tablespoon): 53 calories; 1 g protein; 5 g total fat; 1 g saturated fat; 1 g carbohydrates; 0 g fibre; 158 mg sodium

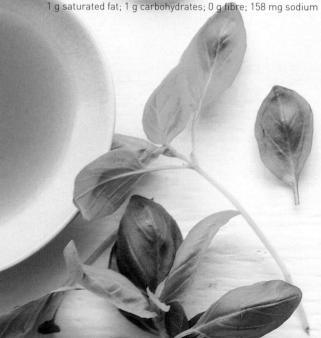

Basil Pesto

2 handfuls of basil leaves, rinsed and dried
2 tablespoons garlic-infused olive oil
2 tablespoons olive oil, plus more as needed
50 g pine nuts
25 g grated Parmesan
Salt and freshly ground black pepper

Combine the basil, garlic-infused oil, olive oil, pine nuts and Parmesan in a food processor or blender and process until well combined. Season to taste with salt and pepper. Add more oil if you prefer a more liquid pesto for drizzling. Spoon into a bowl or jar and cover with a thin layer of olive oil. Cover and store in the fridge for up to 5 days or in the freezer for up to 2 months.

PER SERVING (1 tablespoon): 107 calories; 3 g protein; 10 g total fat; 2 g saturated fat; 1 g carbohydrates; 0 g fibre; 102 mg sodium

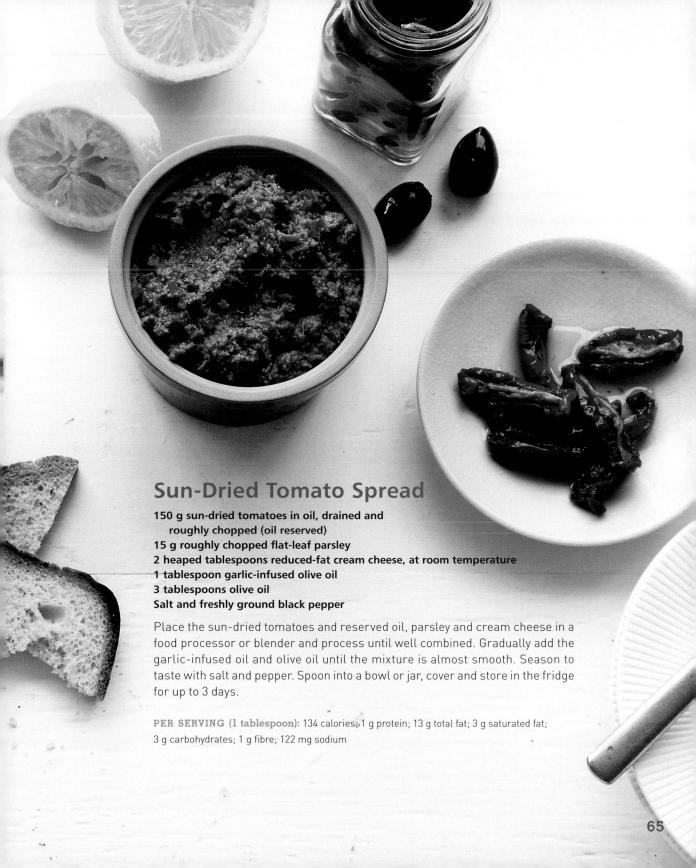

Sun-Dried Tomato Spread

150 g sun-dried tomatoes in oil, drained and
  roughly chopped (oil reserved)
15 g roughly chopped flat-leaf parsley
2 heaped tablespoons reduced-fat cream cheese, at room temperature
1 tablespoon garlic-infused olive oil
3 tablespoons olive oil
Salt and freshly ground black pepper

Place the sun-dried tomatoes and reserved oil, parsley and cream cheese in a
food processor or blender and process until well combined. Gradually add the
garlic-infused oil and olive oil until the mixture is almost smooth. Season to
taste with salt and pepper. Spoon into a bowl or jar, cover and store in the fridge
for up to 3 days.

PER SERVING (1 tablespoon): 134 calories; 1 g protein; 13 g total fat; 3 g saturated fat;
3 g carbohydrates; 1 g fibre; 122 mg sodium

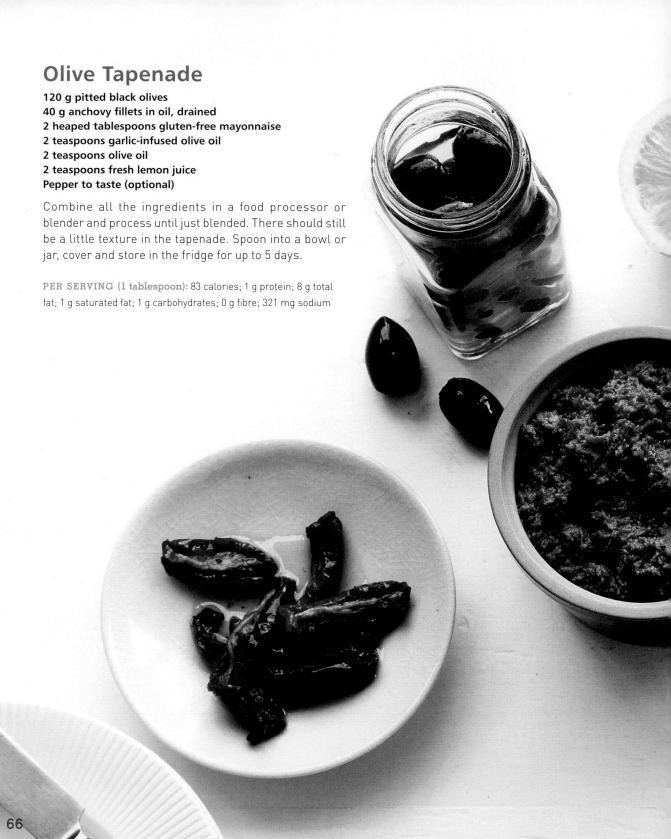

Olive Tapenade

120 g pitted black olives
40 g anchovy fillets in oil, drained
2 heaped tablespoons gluten-free mayonnaise
2 teaspoons garlic-infused olive oil
2 teaspoons olive oil
2 teaspoons fresh lemon juice
Pepper to taste (optional)

Combine all the ingredients in a food processor or blender and process until just blended. There should still be a little texture in the tapenade. Spoon into a bowl or jar, cover and store in the fridge for up to 5 days.

PER SERVING (1 tablespoon): 83 calories; 1 g protein; 8 g total fat; 1 g saturated fat; 1 g carbohydrates; 0 g fibre; 321 mg sodium

Spinach and Pepper Salad with Fried Tofu Puffs

SERVES 4

This is a salad with an Asian twist. Use a light hand with the sesame oil in the dressing; otherwise, its flavour can be a little overpowering. You may be able to find fried tofu puffs in the refrigerator section of Asian supermarkets; otherwise, make your own by frying pressed, cubed extra firm tofu in hot oil.

1. Combine the soy sauce, lemon juice, vinegar, brown sugar and sesame oil in a small bowl and whisk well.

2. Toss the spinach, pea shoots, pepper, tofu and pine nuts in a large bowl until well combined. Drizzle with the dressing and toss briefly. Season to taste with salt and pepper and serve.

PER SERVING: 571 calories; 24 g protein; 40 g total fat; 6 g saturated fat; 40 g carbohydrates; 9 g fibre; 1054 mg sodium

60 ml gluten-free soy sauce

60 ml fresh lemon juice

1 tablespoon plus 1 teaspoon seasoned rice vinegar

55 g light brown sugar

60 ml sesame oil

300 g baby spinach leaves, rinsed and dried

75 g pea shoots or bean sprouts

1 green pepper, seeded and sliced

400 g fried tofu puffs, cut into cubes

50 g pine nuts

Salt and freshly ground black pepper

Peppered Beef and Citrus Salad

SERVES 4

You can make this refreshing salad either with pan-fried beef, as noted in the recipe, or with leftover beef from last night's roast (in which case you can skip the first step).

1. Heat the olive oil in a frying pan over medium heat. Add the beef and cook for 4 minutes on each side for medium-rare, or to your preferred doneness. Let the beef rest for 10 minutes, then slice it thinly.

2. Make the marinade by whisking together the garlic-infused oil, pepper, lemon juice, brown sugar and salt to taste in a medium bowl. Add the beef and toss until well coated in the marinade. Cover and refrigerate for 3 hours.

3. Combine the orange segments, lettuce, water chestnuts, beef and any remaining marinade in a large bowl. Finish with several grinds of black pepper and serve immediately.

PER SERVING: 369 calories; 23 g protein; 23 g total fat; 8 g saturated fat; 18 g carbohydrates; 4 g fibre; 361 mg sodium

2 teaspoons olive oil

450 g beef sirloin or top round steak

2 teaspoons garlic-infused olive oil

1 heaped tablespoon freshly ground black pepper, plus more for serving

60 ml fresh lemon juice

1 heaped tablespoon light brown sugar

Salt

1 orange, peeled and cut into segments

1 head butter lettuce (Boston or Bibb), leaves separated

One 225-g tin water chestnuts, drained and roughly chopped

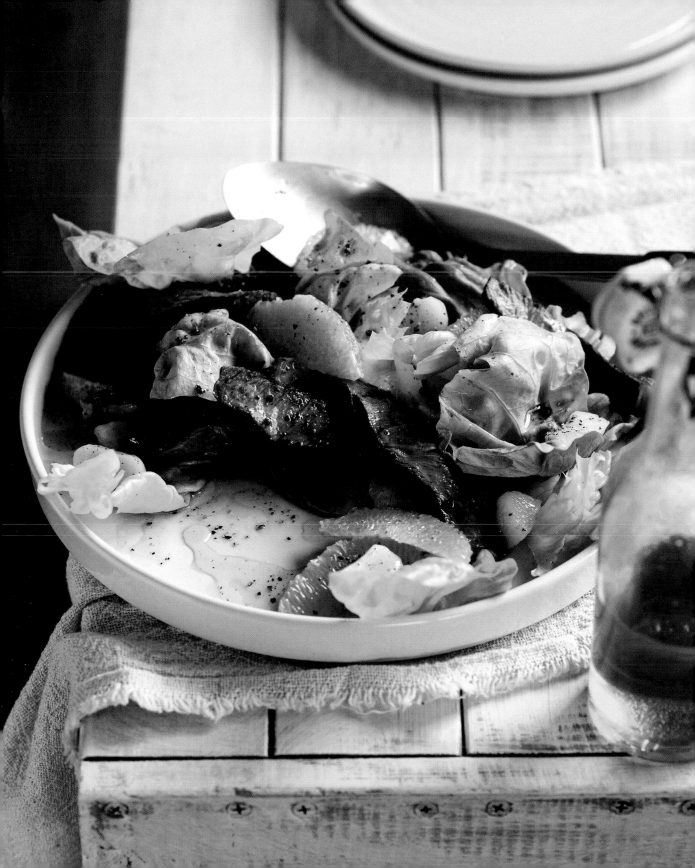

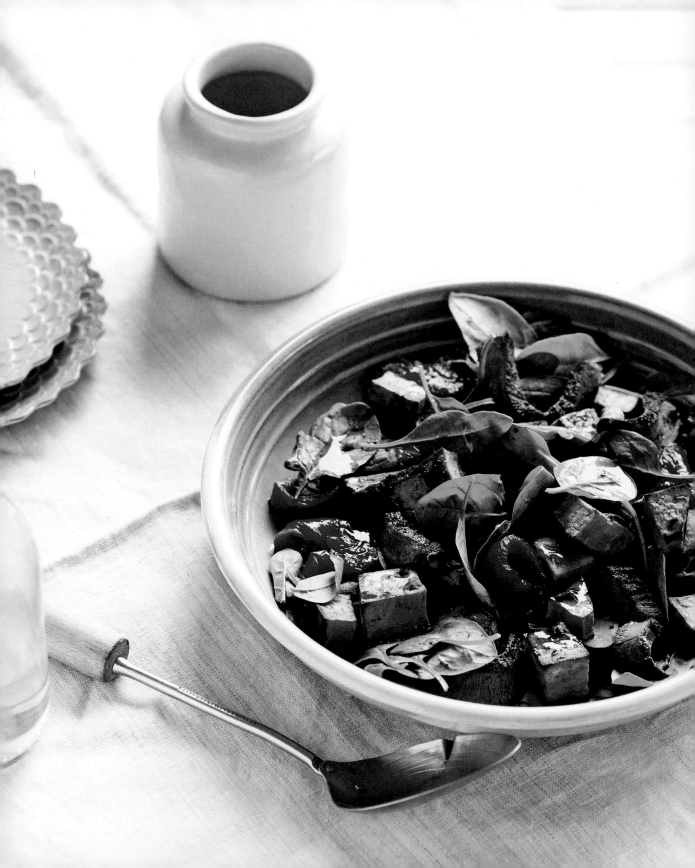

Roasted Sweet Potato Salad with Spiced Lamb and Spinach

SERVES 4

The lamb in this simple salad is flavoured with fragrant Middle Eastern spices, and the vibrant colours of the accompanying vegetables look striking on the plate.

1. Preheat the oven to 180°C.

2. Place the sweet potato and red pepper on a large baking sheet and brush with olive oil. Roast for 30 minutes or until tender and browned. Set aside to cool. When cool enough to handle, remove the skin from the pepper.

3. Heat a little olive oil in a medium frying pan over medium-low heat. Add the cumin, coriander, cardamom, turmeric and sumac and heat for 1 minute or until fragrant. Add the lamb and stir to coat with the spice mix. Cook for 3 to 5 minutes, until just browned. Remove from the heat.

4. Combine the spinach, sweet potato and red pepper in a large bowl. Top with the lamb and any pan juices and finish with a drizzle of olive oil.

PER SERVING: 392 calories; 27 g protein; 14 g total fat; 3 g saturated fat; 40 g carbohydrates; 8 g fibre; 171 mg sodium

4 small sweet potatoes, peeled (if desired) and cut into 2-cm cubes (about 600 g)

1 red pepper, seeded and cut into quarters

Olive oil

1 heaped tablespoon ground cumin

2 teaspoons ground coriander

½ teaspoon ground cardamom

2 teaspoons ground turmeric

½ teaspoon ground sumac, or ½ teaspoon paprika plus ½ teaspoon lemon zest

450 g lean lamb steak, cut into thin strips

225 g baby spinach leaves, rinsed and dried

Caramelised Squash Salad with Sun-Dried Tomatoes and Basil

SERVES 4

Soft, caramelised roasted winter squash is a favourite for many. Balanced with the intense flavours of sun-dried tomato and fresh basil, this salad makes a hearty meat-free lunch. Sprinkle walnuts or pumpkin seeds over the top for crunch and extra nutrition.

1. Preheat the oven to 180°C.
2. Spread the squash and aubergine on two separate baking sheets and brush with 2 tablespoons of the olive oil. Bake for 25 minutes or until tender and golden brown. Let cool to room temperature, then roughly chop the aubergine.
3. Combine the squash, aubergine, sun-dried tomatoes, corn, basil and the remaining 2 tablespoons of olive oil in a large bowl. Refrigerate for 2 to 3 hours to allow the flavours to develop. Bring to room temperature before serving.

PER SERVING: 288 calories; 5 g protein; 15 g total fat; 2 g saturated fat; 41 g carbohydrates; 8 g fibre; 148 mg sodium

1.2 kg kabocha or other suitable winter squash, peeled, seeded, and cut into 2-cm cubes

1 aubergine, cut into 5-mm slices

60 ml olive oil

12 or 13 pieces (50 g) sun-dried tomatoes in oil, drained and sliced

100 g thawed frozen sweetcorn

Small handful of basil leaves, roughly chopped

Blue Cheese and Rocket Salad with Red Wine Dressing

SERVES 4

The combination of blue cheese, rocket and red wine vinegar works beautifully in this salad, giving it a good bite. It works particularly well with grilled or roasted red meat or chicken.

1. Combine the rocket, pea shoots, blue cheese, cucumber, avocado (if using) and green pepper in a large bowl.

2. To make the dressing, combine all the ingredients in a small screw-top jar and shake until well mixed.

3. Just before serving, pour the dressing over the salad and gently toss to combine.

PER SERVING: 403 calories; 13 g protein; 36 g total fat; 3 g saturated fat; 12 g carbohydrates; 4 g fibre; 728 mg sodium

4 handfuls of rocket

50 g pea shoots or bean sprouts

200 g blue cheese, cut into small chunks

½ cucumber, sliced

1 avocado, pitted, peeled and sliced (optional)

½ green pepper, seeded and thinly sliced

RED WINE DRESSING

60 ml olive oil

2 tablespoons plus 2 teaspoons fresh lemon juice

1 tablespoon red wine vinegar

1 teaspoon gluten-free wholegrain mustard

1 teaspoon sugar

2 heaped tablespoons chopped tarragon or flat-leaf parsley

Vietnamese Beef Noodle Salad

SERVES 4

Chinese five-spice powder has a really lovely flavour. Infuse beef with this spice blend and other Asian flavours and see how it sings in this salad. Gluten-free tempeh can also stand in for beef; steam it for 10 minutes, then marinate it for an hour before cooking it as you would the beef.

1. To make the marinade, combine the garlic-infused oil, olive oil, five-spice powder, fish sauce, vinegar, ginger and brown sugar in a medium glass or ceramic bowl. Add the beef strips and toss so the meat is well coated in the marinade. Cover and refrigerate for 3 hours.

2. Fill a large bowl with very hot water. Add the vermicelli and soak for 4 to 5 minutes, until softened. Drain and rinse under cold water, then drain again.

3. Heat the sesame oil in a non-stick frying pan or wok over medium heat. Add the beef strips and any remaining marinade and toss until just cooked through, 2 to 4 minutes. Don't overcook the meat – you want it to be nice and tender.

4. Combine the beef and any juices, vermicelli, pea shoots and mint in a bowl and serve immediately.

PER SERVING: 598 calories; 28 g protein; 28 g total fat; 8 g saturated fat; 50 g carbohydrates; 3 g fibre; 1457 mg sodium

2 teaspoons garlic-infused olive oil

2 teaspoons olive oil

1 heaped tablespoon Chinese five-spice powder

60 ml fish sauce, or 3 tablespoons soy sauce and 1 tablespoon fresh lime juice

60 ml seasoned rice vinegar

2 teaspoons grated ginger

1 heaped tablespoon light brown sugar

450 g beef sirloin or top round steak, cut into thin strips

225 g gluten-free rice vermicelli

2 tablespoons sesame oil

50 g pea shoots or bean sprouts

15 g roughly chopped Vietnamese mint, or a combination of mint and coriander

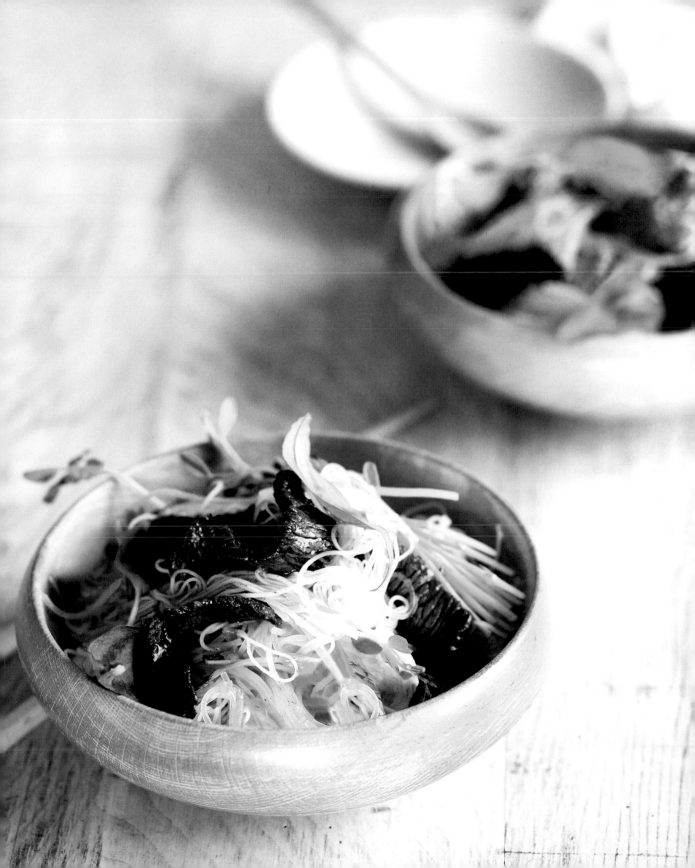

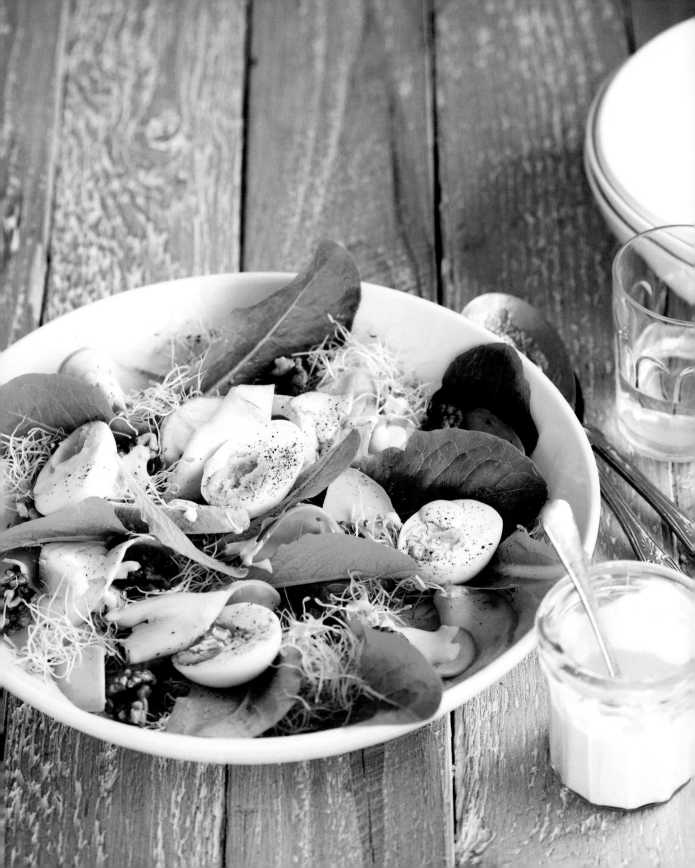

Smoked Chicken and Walnut Salad

SERVES 4

Use smoked chicken if you can find it, because it gives such a wonderful flavour to pasta, sandwiches, wraps and of course salads like this. This dish is perfect to serve when entertaining friends.

1. To make the dressing, whisk together the mayonnaise, soy sauce and lemon juice in a small bowl.

2. Combine the lettuce, sprouts, eggs and avocado (if using) in a large salad bowl. Drizzle the dressing over the top and toss gently to coat. Just before serving, add the chicken and walnuts, season to taste and serve.

PER SERVING: 442 calories; 22 g protein; 36 g total fat; 5 g saturated fat; 8 g carbohydrates; 4 g fibre; 1009 mg sodium

150 g gluten-free mayonnaise

½ teaspoon gluten-free soy sauce

3 tablespoons fresh lemon juice

2 heads baby romaine lettuce, leaves separated

20 g alfalfa sprouts

4 large hard-boiled eggs, halved

1 avocado, pitted, peeled and sliced (optional)

400 g smoked chicken or plain roast chicken, thinly sliced

25 g toasted walnuts

Salt and freshly ground black pepper

Vermicelli Salad with Chicken, Coriander and Mint

SERVES 4–6

You can use leftover roast or rotisserie chicken for this lovely fresh salad, or poach a couple of chicken breasts. To do this, place 2 medium skinless chicken breasts in a small frying pan, cover with water, and simmer gently over medium heat for 12 minutes, turning the chicken halfway through. Remove from the heat, let the chicken cool in the water, then shred the meat. Easy and delicious. Sliced pressed tofu, briefly browned in oil, makes a good vegetarian substitute, if desired.

1. Fill a large bowl with very hot water. Add the vermicelli and soak for 4 to 5 minutes, until softened. Drain and rinse under cold water, then drain again.

2. To make the dressing, combine all the ingredients in a small screw-top jar and shake until well mixed.

3. Combine the noodles, chicken, coriander and mint in a large bowl. Add the dressing, season to taste with salt and pepper and toss well to combine. Refrigerate for 2 to 3 hours before serving to allow the flavours to meld.

PER SERVING (⅙ recipe): 395 calories; 35 g protein; 6 g total fat; 1 g saturated fat; 42 g carbohydrates; 2 g fibre; 406 mg sodium

300 g gluten-free rice vermicelli

350 g shredded cooked chicken breasts

Small handful of coriander leaves, roughly chopped

Small handful of mint leaves, roughly chopped

Salt and freshly ground black pepper

DRESSING

2 tablespoons fresh lime juice

1 tablespoon fish sauce, or 2 teaspoons soy sauce and 1 extra teaspoon fresh lime juice

2 tablespoons light brown sugar

½ red chilli pepper, seeded and finely chopped

1 tablespoon sesame oil

Vegetable Soup

SERVES 4–6

There is a whole lot of goodness in each bowl of this tasty soup. You can add any other low-FODMAP vegetables you happen to have – a great way to make sure they don't go to waste.

1. Heat the oil in a large heavy-bottomed stockpot over medium heat. Add the celery and cook, stirring, until golden brown. Add the broccoli, swede, carrots, squash and potatoes. Pour in the stock. Bring to a boil, reduce the heat, and simmer, covered, for 1 hour or until the vegetables are tender.

2. Remove from the heat and leave to cool to room temperature. Use an immersion blender to purée the vegetables to a smooth consistency. (Alternatively, carefully transfer the vegetables to a food processor and process until smooth.)

3. Stir in the milk, season to taste with salt and pepper and reheat gently.

PER SERVING (⅙ recipe): 231 calories; 10 g protein; 6 g total fat; 1 g saturated fat; 39 g carbohydrates; 12 g fibre; 579 mg sodium

---

* Most stocks contain onion or garlic. Choose one that is onion-free. If garlic is present, the amount is likely to be minimal and should be suitable for most people on a low-FODMAP diet. If you are extremely sensitive to garlic, replace the stock with water, or make your own stock by boiling suitable vegetables (including carrot and celery) in water with your choice of seasonings for about an hour, then straining out the solids.

2 tablespoons garlic-infused olive oil

2 celery stalks, tough strings removed, halved lengthwise and cut into 5-mm slices

1 head broccoli, cut into chunks (including stalks)

3 swede, peeled and cut into chunks

2 large carrots, cut into chunks

400 g kabocha or other suitable winter squash, peeled, seeded and cut into chunks

3 potatoes, cut into chunks

1 litre gluten-free, onion-free vegetable stock*

375 ml semi-skimmed milk, lactose-free milk or suitable plant-based milk

Salt and freshly ground black pepper

Spicy Clear Soup

SERVES 4

Galangal root (an optional but highly recommended addition to this recipe) is available bottled or frozen in Asian grocers and sometimes fresh in the produce section of some supermarkets. If you are using dried galangal, soak it in boiling water until softened before proceeding with the recipe. Even without the galangal, this soup is light and flavourful.

1. Heat the sesame oil, garlic-infused oil and rice bran oil in a large saucepan over medium heat. Add the lemongrass and red chilli and cook for 2 minutes or until fragrant.

2. Add the galangal (if using), stock, fish sauce and lime juice and bring to a boil. Add the bok choy, coriander, bamboo shoots, baby corn and vermicelli. Reduce the heat and simmer for 3 minutes or until the vegetables and noodles are tender. (Remove the galangal.) Serve immediately.

PER SERVING: 227 calories; 7 g protein; 8 g total fat; 1 g saturated fat; 28 g carbohydrates; 4 g fibre; 1671 mg sodium

---

* Most stocks contain onion or garlic. Choose one that is onion-free. If garlic is present, the amount is likely to be minimal and should be suitable for most people on a low-FODMAP diet. If you are extremely sensitive to garlic, replace the stock with water and double the quantities of sesame oil, lemongrass, fish sauce, lime juice and coriander, or make your own stock by boiling chicken bones and/or suitable vegetables (including carrot and celery) in water with your choice of seasonings for about an hour, then straining out the solids.

1 tablespoon sesame oil

2 teaspoons garlic-infused olive oil

2 teaspoons rice bran oil or sunflower oil

2 heaped tablespoons finely chopped lemongrass (white portion only)

½ to 1 red chilli seeded and finely chopped

6 pieces dried galangal root (optional)

1.5 litres gluten-free, onion-free chicken or vegetable stock*

2 tablespoons plus 2 teaspoons fish sauce, or 4 teaspoons soy sauce and 2 teaspoons fresh lime juice

1 tablespoon plus 1 teaspoon fresh lime juice

3 bunches baby bok choy, quartered, rinsed and drained

2 heaped tablespoons chopped coriander

One 225-g tin bamboo shoots, drained

One 400-g tin baby corn, drained, or 215 g fresh baby corn, cut on the diagonal

100 g gluten-free rice vermicelli

Chicken Noodle Soup with Bok Choy

SERVES 4

I really enjoy the ginger and lime in this soup. Please use the quantities as a guide – you can certainly increase the amounts I suggest in the recipe. I often do!

1. Place the stock, ginger and lime leaves in a large heavy-bottomed saucepan and bring to a boil. Add the chicken, reduce the heat and simmer for 5 minutes.

2. Add the rice noodles, bok choy and bean sprouts and simmer for another 5 minutes or until the noodles are tender. Remove the lime leaves, stir in the soy sauce and serve immediately.

PER SERVING: 362 calories; 31 g protein; 2 g total fat; 0 g saturated fat; 46 g carbohydrates; 2 g fibre; 1023 mg sodium

---

* Most stocks contain onion or garlic. Choose one that is onion-free. If garlic is present, the amount is likely to be minimal and should be suitable for most people on a low-FODMAP diet. If you are extremely sensitive to garlic, omit the stock and use water instead, or make your own stock by boiling chicken bones and/or suitable vegetables (including carrot and celery) in water with your choice of seasonings for about an hour, then straining out the solids.

2 litres gluten-free, onion-free chicken or vegetable stock*

1 heaped tablespoon grated ginger

4 kaffir lime leaves

450 g boneless, skinless chicken breasts, very thinly sliced

225 g gluten-free rice vermicelli, broken into 5-cm pieces

3 bunches baby bok choy, leaves separated, rinsed and drained

40 g bean sprouts

2 teaspoons gluten-free soy sauce

Curried Potato and Parsnip Soup

SERVES 4

This creamy, comforting soup is perfect for a cold winter's night. The flavour actually improves if left to mature for a day, so try to make it ahead of time if you can.

1. Heat the canola oil in a large heavy-bottomed saucepan over medium heat. Add the parsnips and potatoes and cook, stirring regularly, for 3 to 5 minutes, until lightly golden. Add the stock and bring to a boil. Reduce the heat and simmer for 15 to 20 minutes, stirring occasionally, until the vegetables are tender. Remove from the heat and let cool for about 10 minutes.

2. Purée with an immersion blender (or in batches in a regular blender) until smooth. Add the curry powder and milk and blend again until well combined. Season to taste with salt and pepper. Reheat gently without boiling. Garnish with a sprinkling of parsley and serve.

PER SERVING: 215 calories; 10 g protein; 4 g total fat; 1 g saturated fat; 36 g carbohydrates; 12 g fibre; 766 mg sodium

1 tablespoon canola oil

2 parsnips (400 g), peeled and cut into 2-cm pieces

4 potatoes (800 g), peeled and cut into 2-cm pieces

1.5 litres gluten-free, onion-free chicken or vegetable stock*

1 teaspoon gluten-free curry powder, or to taste

250 ml semi-skimmed milk, lactose-free milk or suitable plant-based milk

Salt and freshly ground black pepper

Chopped flat-leaf parsley, to garnish

---

* Most stocks contain onion or garlic. Choose one that is onion-free. If garlic is present, the amount is likely to be minimal and should be suitable for most people on a low-FODMAP diet. If you are extremely sensitive to garlic, omit the stock and use water instead, or make your own stock by boiling chicken bones and/or suitable vegetables (including carrot and celery) in water with your choice of seasonings for about an hour, then straining out the solids.

Carrot and Ginger Soup

SERVES 6

You won't believe how perfectly the flavours of carrot and ginger complement each other, and the ginger adds a warm twist. Comfort food in a bowl.

1. Heat the olive oil in a large heavy-bottomed saucepan over medium heat, add the celeriac and cook until golden. Add the carrots, potatoes and stock. Bring to a boil, reduce the heat, cover and simmer for 20 minutes or until the vegetables are tender. Let cool for about 10 minutes, then purée with an immersion blender (or in batches in a regular blender) until smooth.

2. Stir in the ginger and milk until well combined. You can adjust the quantity of milk depending on how thick you like your soup. Season to taste with salt and pepper. Reheat gently without boiling and serve.

PER SERVING: 225 calories; 7 g protein; 4 g total fat; 1 g saturated fat; 44 g carbohydrates; 12 g fibre; 713 mg sodium

1 tablespoon olive oil

1 small celeriac (about 400 g), peeled, halved and cut into 5-mm slices

1.8 kg carrots, cut into 2-cm chunks

2 large potatoes (600 g), peeled and cut into quarters

1.5 litres gluten-free, onion-free chicken or vegetable stock*

1 heaped tablespoon ground ginger

250 ml semi-skimmed milk, lactose-free milk or suitable plant-based milk

Salt and freshly ground black pepper

---

* Most stocks contain onion or garlic. Choose one that is onion-free. If garlic is present, the amount is likely to be minimal and should be suitable for most people on a low-FODMAP diet. If you are extremely sensitive to garlic, omit the stock and use water instead, or make your own stock by boiling chicken bones and/or suitable vegetables (including carrot and celery) in water with your choice of seasonings for about an hour, then straining out the solids.

Roasted Squash and Chestnut Soup

SERVES 4

The point of difference in this soup is the chestnut purée. It adds a gorgeous base flavour and is well worth seeking out. Look for it in large supermarkets and gourmet food stores. If necessary, you can make your own by puréeing peeled roasted chestnuts (available in some supermarkets and Asian grocery stores) in the food processor or blender.

1. Preheat the oven to 180°C.

2. Spread the squash on a baking sheet and drizzle with the olive oil. Bake, turning occasionally, for 30 to 40 minutes, until golden and cooked through.

3. Transfer the squash to a large saucepan or stockpot. Add the chestnut purée, stock and ginger and bring to a boil. Reduce the heat and simmer over medium-low heat for 15 to 20 minutes, stirring occasionally, until the squash is tender. Let cool for about 10 minutes.

4. Add the warmed milk to the soup and purée with an immersion blender (or in batches in a regular blender) until smooth. Season to taste with salt and pepper. Finish with a swirl of extra milk (if desired) and serve.

PER SERVING: 466 calories; 9 g protein; 10 g total fat; 2 g saturated fat; 92 g carbohydrates; 8 g fibre; 928 mg sodium

2 kg peeled, seeded, and cubed kabocha or other suitable winter squash

2 tablespoons olive oil

500 g unsweetened chestnut purée

2 litres gluten-free, onion-free chicken or vegetable stock*

2 teaspoons ground ginger

250 ml semi-skimmed milk, lactose-free milk or suitable plant-based milk, warmed, plus more for serving (optional)

Salt and freshly ground black pepper

---

* Most stocks contain onion or garlic. Choose one that is onion-free. If garlic is present, the amount is likely to be minimal and should be suitable for most people on a low-FODMAP diet. If you are extremely sensitive to garlic, omit the stock and use water instead, or make your own stock by boiling chicken bones and/or suitable vegetables (including carrot and celery) in water with your choice of seasonings for about an hour, then straining out the solids.

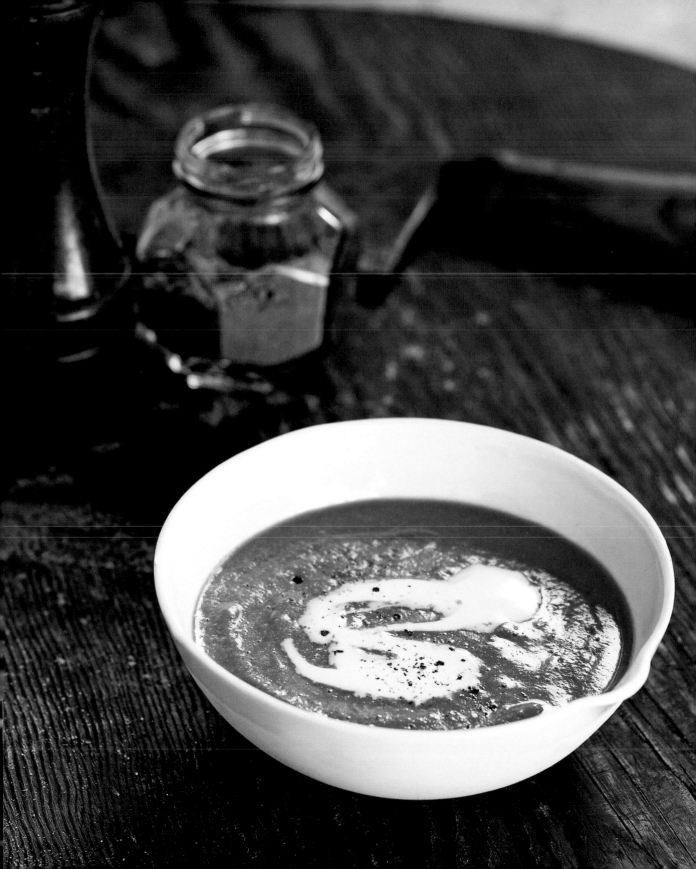

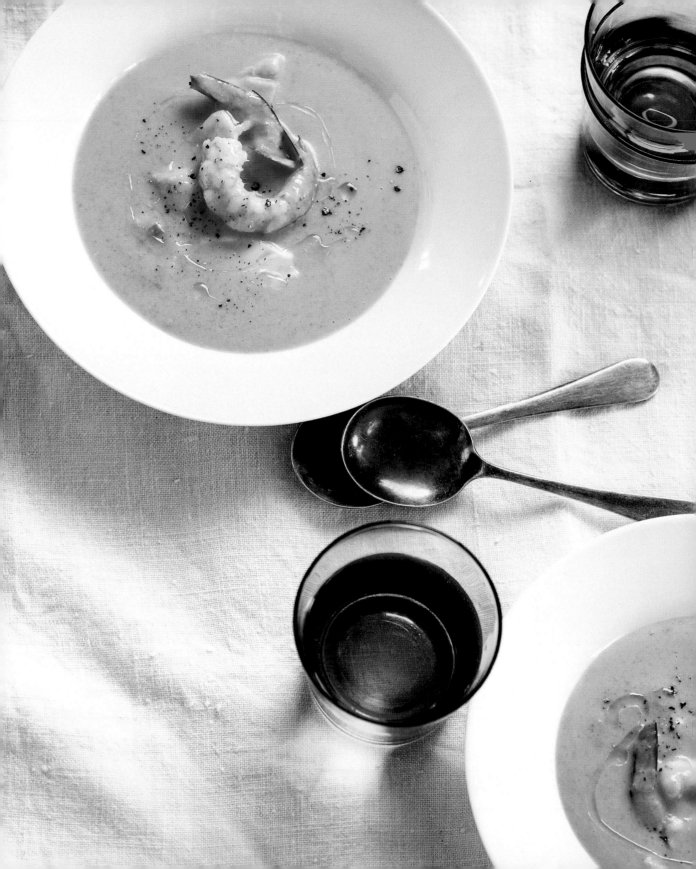

Creamy Seafood Soup

SERVES 6

You can use any combination of seafood in this creamy soup. Although it makes sense to use fish stock in a seafood dish it's very difficult to find one that is onion-free, unless of course it's homemade. For that reason I have suggested chicken stock in the recipe.

1. Melt the butter in a large heavy-bottomed saucepan over medium heat. Add the carrots and rice and cook, stirring regularly, for 5 minutes.

2. Add the stock, fish sauce, tomato passata, fennel and wine (if using) and stir to combine. Bring to a boil, reduce the heat to low and simmer for 20 minutes, until the rice is tender.

3. Let cool for 10 minutes. Purée with an immersion blender (or in batches in a regular blender) until smooth.

4. Return the pan to the stove over medium heat and bring the soup to a simmer. Add the uncooked prawns, squid and fish and simmer for 4 to 5 minutes, until the seafood is just cooked. Add the jumbo prawns and milk and stir until heated through and combined. Season to taste with salt and pepper, finish with a drizzle of olive oil (if desired) and serve immediately.

PER SERVING (with optional wine): 296 calories; 32 g protein; 9 g total fat; 4 g saturated fat; 17 g carbohydrates; 2 g fibre; 1300 mg sodium

---

* Most stocks contain onion or garlic. Choose one that is onion-free. If garlic is present, the amount is likely to be minimal and should be suitable for most people on a low-FODMAP diet. If you are extremely sensitive to garlic, omit the stock and use water instead, or make your own stock by boiling chicken bones and suitable vegetables (including carrot and celery) in water with your choice of seasonings for about an hour, then straining out the solids.

45 g salted butter

2 large carrots, diced

100 g long-grain white rice

1.25 litres gluten-free, onion-free chicken stock*

2 tablespoons plus 2 teaspoons fish sauce, or 4 teaspoons soy sauce plus 2 teaspoons fresh lime juice

125 ml tomato passata

½ fennel bulb, finely chopped

125 ml white wine (optional)

450 g raw medium prawns, peeled and deveined

2 large or 5 small squid bodies, cleaned and sliced (150 g)

150 g boneless, skinless firm fish fillets, cut into cubes

6 cooked jumbo prawns

250 ml semi-skimmed milk, lactose-free milk or suitable plant-based milk

Salt and freshly ground black pepper

Extra virgin olive oil, to garnish (optional)

Mussels in Chilli, Bacon and Tomato Broth

SERVES 4

The addition of bacon and chilli to the tomato broth give this dish lovely smoky background notes with a little zing. You can adjust the zing to your own preference; it certainly still tastes delicious without any cayenne!

1. In a large heavy-bottomed saucepan over medium heat, cook the bacon until just golden. Spoon out and discard any excess fat, then add the olive oil, tomato passata, cayenne and 500 ml of the stock. Bring to a boil, reduce the heat to low and simmer for 30 to 40 minutes to develop the smoky bacon flavour.

2. Add the remaining stock. Increase the heat to medium-high and bring to a boil. Add the mussels and cook, covered, for 5 to 8 minutes, until all the mussels have opened. Shake the pan to redistribute the mussels and cook for an extra minute. Shake again. Discard any unopened mussels. Season to taste with salt and pepper and serve immediately with plenty of gluten-free bread to mop up the delicious broth.

PER SERVING (not including the bread): 612 calories; 59 g protein; 26 g total fat; 7 g saturated fat; 33 g carbohydrates; 4 g fibre; 2082 mg sodium

113 g lean bacon slices, cut crosswise into thin strips

2 tablespoons olive oil

750 ml tomato passata

½ teaspoon cayenne pepper (or to taste)

1.5 litres reduced sodium gluten-free, onion-free chicken stock*

2.5 kg mussels, scrubbed and debearded

Salt and freshly ground black pepper

Gluten-free bread, for serving

---

* Most stocks contain onion or garlic. Choose one that is onion-free. If garlic is present, the amount is likely to be minimal and should be suitable for most people on a low-FODMAP diet. If you are extremely sensitive to garlic, omit the stock and use water mixed with 1 teaspoon fish sauce instead.

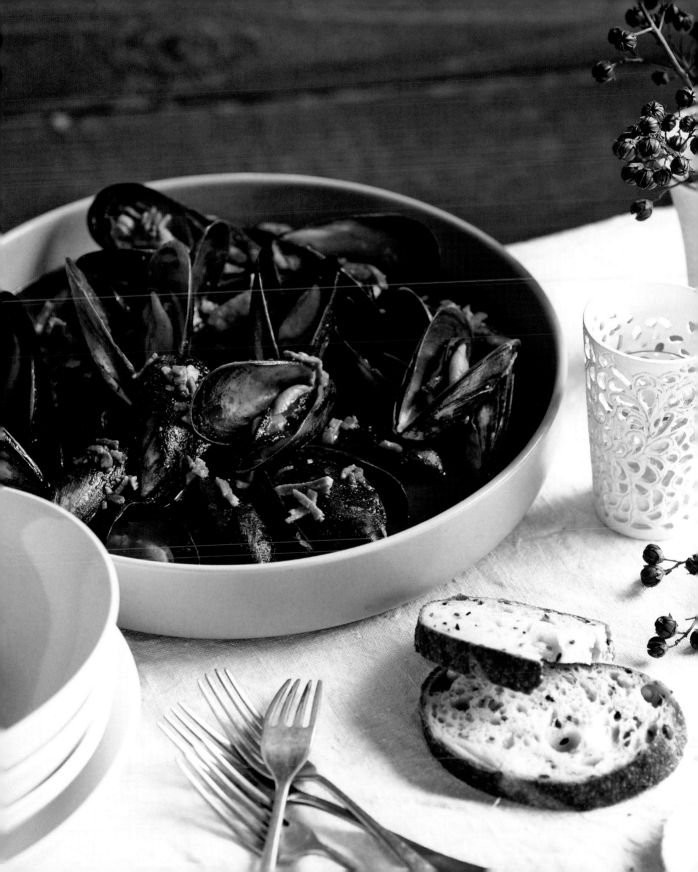

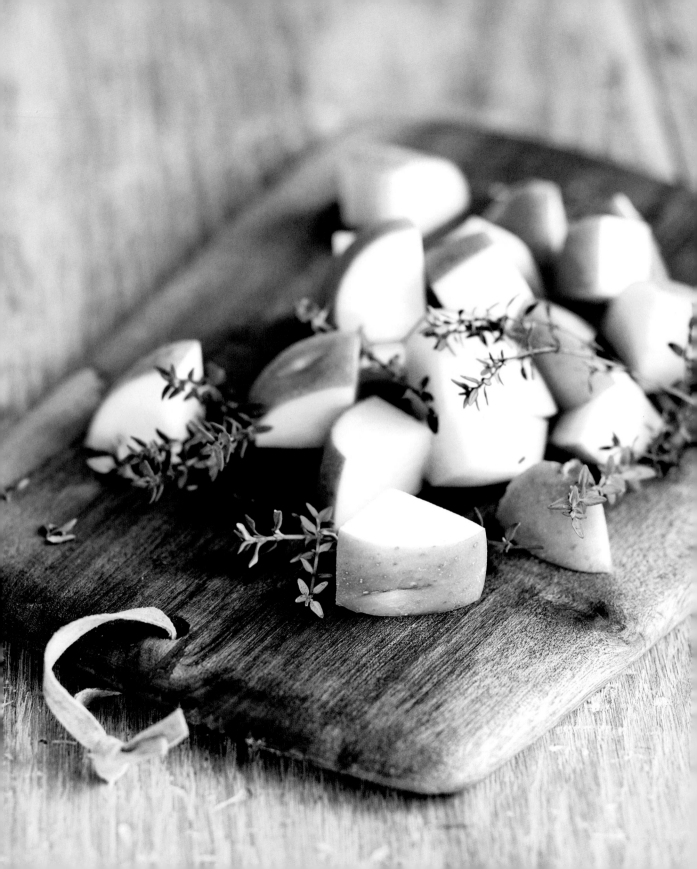

Potato and Corn Chowder

SERVES 6

This hearty soup is really more like a chowder. Smoky bacon and sweetcorn are a classic pairing – although you can leave out the bacon and use vegetable stock to make an equally satisfying vegetarian soup.

1. If using the bacon, add to a large heavy-bottomed saucepan over medium heat and cook, stirring, until crisp. Remove to paper towels to drain. Spray the same saucepan with cooking spray, add the potatoes and cook, still over medium heat, stirring regularly.

2. Pour in the stock and bring to a boil. Reduce the heat to a simmer and cook for 15 minutes, stirring occasionally, until the potatoes are tender.

3. Purée with an immersion blender (or in batches in a regular blender) until smooth. Stir in the sweetcorn, mustard, thyme, parsley and reserved bacon, and season to taste with salt and pepper. Reheat gently without boiling and serve.

PER SERVING (including bacon): 283 calories; 18 g protein; 15 g total fat; 6 g saturated fat; 18 g carbohydrates; 3 g fibre; 1148 mg sodium

---

* Most stocks contain onion or garlic. Choose one that is onion-free. If garlic is present, the amount is likely to be minimal and should be suitable for most people on a low-FODMAP diet. If you are extremely sensitive to garlic, omit the stock and use water instead, or make your own stock by boiling chicken bones and/or suitable vegetables (including carrot and celery) in water with your choice of seasonings for about an hour, then straining out the solids.

225 g lean bacon slices, diced (optional)

Non-stick cooking spray

3 large potatoes, peeled (if desired) and diced

2 litres reduced sodium gluten-free, onion-free chicken or vegetable stock*

One 417-g tin no-salt-added, gluten-free cream-style sweetcorn

1 teaspoon ground mustard

1 teaspoon fresh thyme leaves

1 heaped tablespoon roughly chopped flat-leaf parsley

Salt and freshly ground black pepper

Hearty Lamb Shank and Vegetable Soup

SERVES 4

Hands down, this is my favourite soup, and I think you'll love it, too. Squash forms the base of this thick, hearty soup. If you prefer a meatier flavour, increase the quantity of lamb shanks.

1. Heat the olive oil and garlic-infused oil in a large heavy-bottomed saucepan over medium heat. Add the lamb shanks and cook on all sides until lightly browned, 5 to 10 minutes total, searing for 2 to 3 minutes on each side before turning. Remove the shanks and set aside on a plate. Add the squash, carrots and celery to the pan and cook in the remaining oil and meat juices for 2 to 3 minutes, until lightly golden.

2. Increase the heat to medium-high and return the shanks to the pan. Add the stock and rice and bring to a boil, then reduce the heat and simmer, stirring occasionally, for 50 to 60 minutes, until the meat is very tender.

3. Remove the lamb shanks, then remove the meat from the bones and shred or cut into large pieces. Discard the bones and fat. Return the lamb to the pan and stir until well combined, breaking up the squash pieces. Season well with salt and pepper and serve.

PER SERVING: 623 calories; 40 g protein; 30 g total fat; 8 g saturated fat; 49 g carbohydrates; 5 g fibre; 804 mg sodium

3 tablespoons olive oil

1 tablespoon garlic-infused olive oil

2 lamb shanks (about 900 g)

700 g kabocha or other suitable winter squash, peeled, seeded and cut into 2-cm pieces

3 large carrots, cut into 1-cm pieces

3 celery stalks, cut into 1-cm slices

1.5 litres gluten-free, onion-free beef stock*

130 g long-grain white rice

Salt and freshly ground black pepper

---

* Most stocks contain onion or garlic. Choose one that is onion-free. If garlic is present, the amount is likely to be minimal and should be suitable for most people on a low-FODMAP diet. If you are extremely sensitive to garlic, omit the stock and use water instead, or make your own stock by boiling chicken bones and/or suitable vegetables (including carrot and celery) in water with your choice of seasonings for about an hour, then straining out the solids.

MAINS

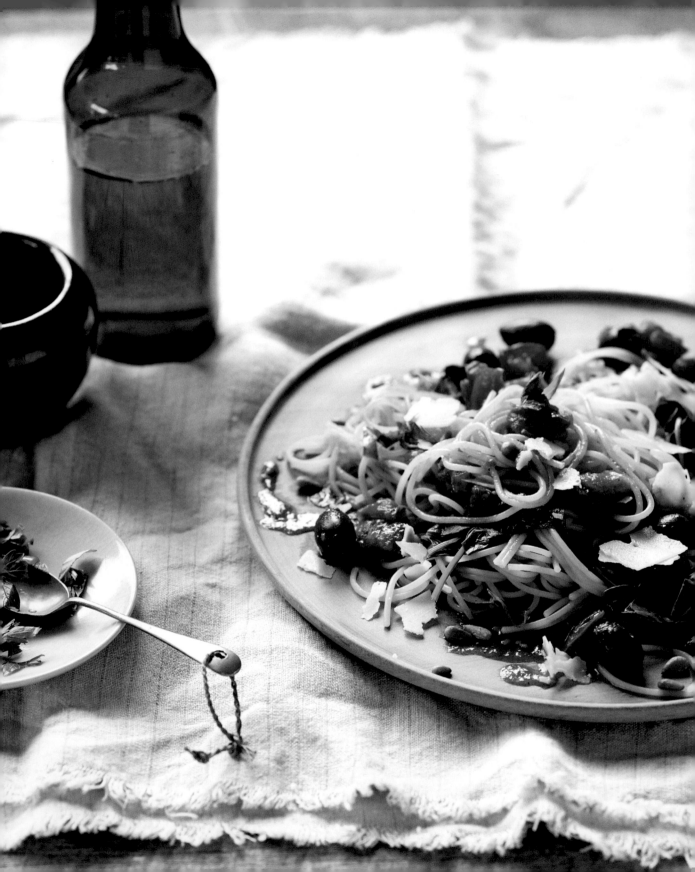

Pasta with Fresh Tomato, Olives and Pecorino

SERVES 4–6

This is a lovely summery pasta dish. Toss together the light Mediterranean flavours of tomatoes, olives, basil and pecorino, and enjoy.

1. Bring a large pot of water to a boil. Add the pasta and cook according to packet directions until just tender. Drain, return to the pot and cover to keep warm.

2. Heat the olive oil in a large heavy-bottomed saucepan over medium heat, add the pine nuts and toss until golden. Add the spinach, olives, tomatoes, basil and parsley and cook until the spinach has wilted.

3. Add the pecorino and heat until warmed through and slightly melted. Season to taste with salt and pepper, add the drained pasta and toss to combine. Serve garnished with extra pecorino.

PER SERVING (⅙ recipe): 452 calories; 13 g protein; 16 g total fat; 1 g saturated fat; 64 g carbohydrates; 3 g fibre; 525 mg sodium

450 g gluten-free pasta

2 tablespoons olive oil

40 g pine nuts

120 g baby spinach leaves, rinsed and dried

160 g kalamata olives, pitted

6 Roma (plum) tomatoes, chopped

5 g basil leaves

15 g flat-leaf parsley leaves

70 g pecorino, shaved, plus more for serving

Salt and freshly ground black pepper

Creamy Blue Cheese and Spinach Pasta

SERVES 4–6

Blue cheese is lactose-free, so this stunning pasta is fine for people with lactose intolerance, as the amount of cream used is minimal.

1. Bring a large pot of water to a boil. Add the pasta and cook according to packet directions, until just tender. Drain, return to the pot and cover to keep warm.

2. Meanwhile, heat the olive oil and garlic-infused oil in a large heavy-bottomed frying pan over medium heat. Add the cream and wine and simmer, stirring occasionally, for 5 to 7 minutes, until the liquid has reduced and thickened. Add the blue cheese and stir until melted.

3. Remove the pan from the heat. Add the drained pasta, spinach and parsley and gently toss to coat. Allow the spinach leaves to wilt. Season to taste with salt and pepper and serve.

PER SERVING (⅙ recipe): 367 calories; 9 g protein; 9 g total fat; 2 g saturated fat; 58 g carbohydrates; 2 g fibre; 343 mg sodium

450 g gluten-free pasta

1 tablespoon olive oil

2 teaspoons garlic-infused olive oil

80 ml single cream

80 ml white wine

35 g crumbled blue cheese

105 g baby spinach leaves, rinsed and dried

15 g roughly chopped flat-leaf parsley

Salt and freshly ground black pepper

Speedy Spaghetti Bolognese

SERVES 6–8

Most recipes for spaghetti Bolognese start with peeling, slicing and dicing an onion, but not this one. Instead, I use bacon to add another dimension to every mouthful. You're going to love it!

1. Bring a large pot of water to a boil. Add the spaghetti and cook according to packet directions, until just tender. Drain, return to the pot and cover to keep warm.

2. Meanwhile, heat the olive oil and garlic-infused oil in a large heavy-bottomed frying pan over medium heat. Add the beef and bacon and cook until the beef is nicely browned, breaking up any lumps as you go. Add the tomato passata, cayenne and chilli powder (if using) and simmer for 10 minutes, stirring occasionally. Season to taste with salt and pepper.

3. Divide the spaghetti among four bowls and spoon the Bolognese sauce over each. Garnish with Parmesan and serve immediately.

PER SERVING (⅛ recipe, not including the Parmesan): 717 calories; 42 g protein; 224 g total fat; 10 g saturated fat; 74 g carbohydrates; 6 g fibre; 925 mg sodium

Two 350-g or three 225-g packets gluten-free spaghetti

2 teaspoons olive oil

2 teaspoons garlic-infused olive oil

900 g extra-lean minced beef

225 g lean bacon slices, diced

670 ml tomato passata

2 teaspoons cayenne pepper

½ teaspoon chilli powder (optional)

Salt and freshly ground black pepper

Grated Parmesan, for serving

Penne with Meatballs

SERVES 6

These meatballs are an excellent way to use up leftover rice, but if you are cooking the rice from scratch, you'll need about 65 g of uncooked rice. If you have any children hovering about in the kitchen, I am sure they will enjoy making this recipe with you.

1. Bring a large pot of water to a boil.

2. To make the meatballs, combine the beef, rice, Parmesan, egg, garlic-infused oil, olive oil, finely chopped basil and parsley, cayenne and salt and pepper in a large bowl. With wet hands, shape into golf ball–size balls.

3. Heat the olive oil in a large frying pan over medium heat, add the meatballs and cook until nicely browned on all sides and cooked through.

4. Meanwhile, add the pasta to the boiling water and cook according to packet directions until just tender. Drain, return to the pot and cover to keep warm.

5. Pour the tomato passata over the meatballs and sprinkle on the roughly chopped basil. Bring to a boil, then reduce the heat and simmer for 2 to 3 minutes, until warmed through.

6. Divide the penne among four bowls and spoon the meatballs and sauce over the top. Garnish with a sprinkling of Parmesan and extra basil leaves, if desired, and serve immediately.

PER SERVING (not including the Parmesan or extra basil): 754 calories; 46 g protein; 24 g total fat; 7 g saturated fat; 82 g carbohydrates; 6 g fibre; 544 mg sodium

MEATBALLS

900 g extra-lean minced beef

220 g cooked long-grain rice

60 g grated Parmesan

1 large egg, beaten

2 teaspoons garlic-infused olive oil

2 teaspoons olive oil

3 to 4 heaped tablespoons finely chopped basil

15 g finely chopped flat-leaf parsley

½ teaspoon cayenne pepper

Salt and freshly ground black pepper

Olive oil, for pan-frying

510 g gluten-free penne

500 ml tomato passata

5 g roughly chopped basil

Grated Parmesan, for serving

Extra basil leaves, for serving (optional)

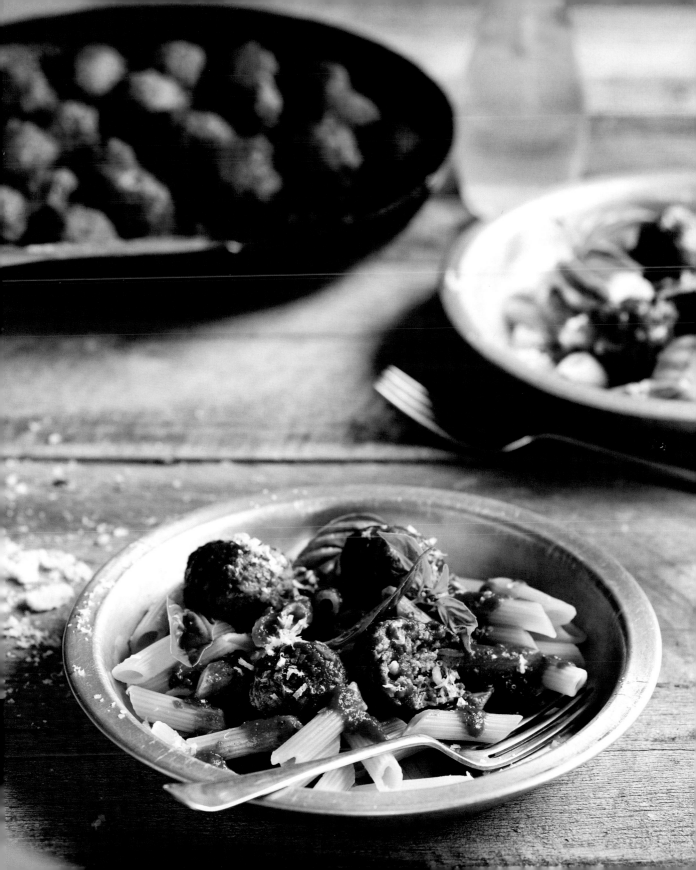

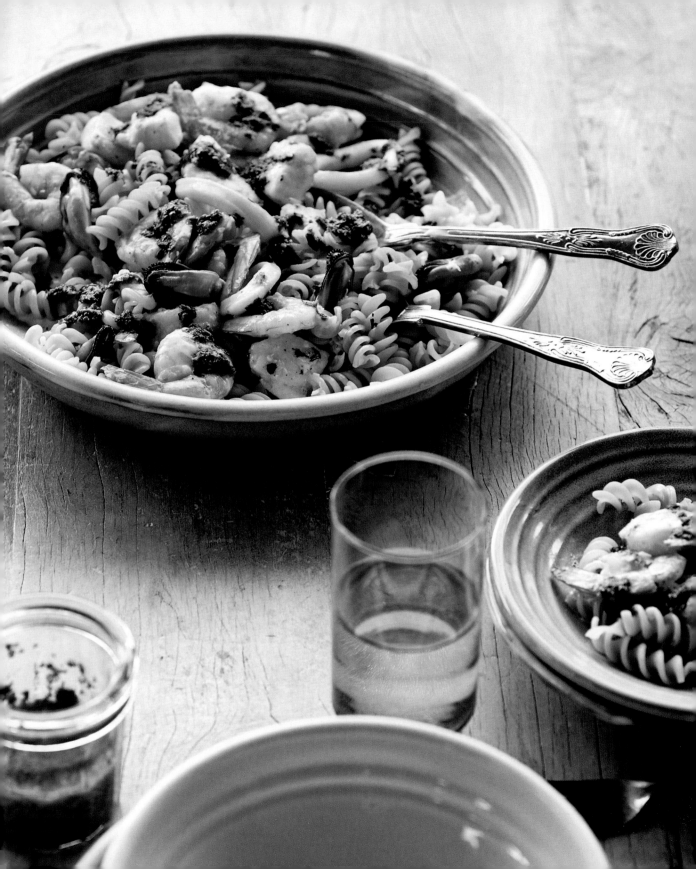

Seafood Pasta with Salsa Verde

SERVES 4

This is a tasty combination of seafood, although you can mix and match with others if you like. Regardless, if possible, always purchase fresh seafood on the day you are making the dish for maximum freshness.

1. Bring a large pot of water to a boil. Add the pasta and cook according to packet directions, until just tender. Drain and return to the pot. Stir in most of the Salsa Verde, cover and keep warm.

2. Meanwhile, heat the olive oil and garlic-infused oil in a large non-stick frying pan over medium-high heat. Add the squid, fish and prawns and cook for 2 minutes, tossing gently. Stir in the mussel meat, cream and wine, reduce the heat and simmer for 3 to 4 minutes, until all the seafood is lightly cooked through. Season to taste with salt and pepper.

3. Divide the pasta among four bowls and spoon the seafood sauce over each. Finish with small dollops of the remaining Salsa Verde and serve immediately.

PER SERVING: 862 calories; 63 g protein; 23 g total fat; 6 g saturated fat; 92 g carbohydrates; 2 g fibre; 958 mg sodium

450 g gluten-free pasta

130 g Salsa Verde (page 64)

2 teaspoons olive oil

2 teaspoons garlic-infused olive oil

2 small squid bodies, cleaned and sliced into rings

225 g boneless, skinless firm white fish fillets, cut into cubes

450 g raw large prawns, peeled and deveined, tails intact

450 g fresh shelled mussel meats

125 ml single cream

2 tablespoons plus 2 teaspoons dry white wine

Salt and freshly ground black pepper

Smoked Chicken Pasta

SERVES 4–6

This light pasta dish has no sauce as such. Instead, sautéed ingredients are stirred into the warm pasta. It's a great introduction to smoked chicken if you haven't tried it before (though the recipe is tasty with plain roast chicken, too).

1. Bring a large pot of water to a boil. Add the pasta and cook according to packet directions, until just tender. Drain and return to the pot. Stir in 2 tablespoons of the olive oil, cover and keep warm.

2. Heat the garlic-infused oil and the remaining 2 tablespoons olive oil in a large frying pan. Add the chicken, spinach and pine nuts and cook, stirring, until the spinach has wilted and the chicken and pine nuts are golden brown. Add the drained pasta and Parmesan and toss over medium heat until the cheese has melted. Season to taste with salt and pepper and finish with an extra drizzle of garlic-infused oil, if desired.

PER SERVING (⅙ recipe): 479 calories; 20 g protein; 17 g total fat; 2 g saturated fat; 58 g carbohydrates; 2 g fibre; 592 mg sodium

450 g gluten-free pasta

60 ml extra virgin olive oil

2 teaspoons garlic-infused olive oil, plus more for serving (optional)

285 g boneless, skinless smoked chicken breast or plain roast chicken breast, sliced

2 large handfuls of baby spinach leaves, rinsed and dried

50 g pine nuts

40 g grated Parmesan

Salt and freshly ground black pepper

Smoked Salmon Pasta in White Wine Sauce

SERVES 4

At last, a creamy pasta we can all enjoy! The garlic is used only to infuse the sauce with flavour and should be well tolerated; be sure to remember to remove it, though.

1. Bring a large pot of water to a boil. Add the pasta and cook according to packet directions, until just tender. Drain, return to the pot and cover to keep warm.

2. Meanwhile, combine the olive oil, wine and garlic in a large frying pan and bring to a boil over high heat, stirring constantly. Reduce the heat to medium and simmer, stirring occasionally, for 5 to 6 minutes, until the sauce has thickened slightly. Remove from the heat and remove and discard the garlic. Add the Parmesan, parsley, pepper and lemon zest and stir until the cheese has melted.

3. Add the sauce and smoked salmon to the pasta and toss to combine. Season to taste with salt and pepper and serve.

PER SERVING: 619 calories; 21 g protein; 20 g total fat; 3 g saturated fat; 85 g carbohydrates; 2 g fibre; 673 mg sodium

450 g gluten-free pasta

60 ml olive oil

125 ml dry white wine

1 garlic clove, peeled and halved

60 g grated Parmesan

20 g roughly chopped flat-leaf parsley

1 teaspoon freshly ground black pepper, plus more if needed

1 teaspoon finely grated lemon zest

113 g smoked salmon, cut into thin strips

Salt

Vegetable Pasta Bake

SERVES 6–8

Gluten-free pasta is available in most supermarkets nowadays, and you can also find it in health food shops. As the pasta is cooked a second time in this recipe, make sure you boil it until it is just barely tender, then rinse it in cold water to stop the residual heat from cooking it further.

1. Begin bringing two large pots of water to a boil. Preheat the oven to 180°C. Grease a 2-litre baking dish with cooking spray.

2. Add the pasta to one pot and cook according to packet directions until just barely tender. Drain and rinse under cold water. Drain again.

3. Meanwhile, add the squash to the other pot and boil until just tender. Drain and set aside.

4. Combine the breadcrumbs and cheddar and set aside.

5. Combine the pasta, squash, tomatoes, courgette, eggs, Parmesan, parsley, cumin and mustard in a large bowl. Season to taste with salt and pepper. Spoon into the baking dish and sprinkle the cheddar and breadcrumbs over the top. Bake for 30 minutes or until golden.

PER SERVING (⅛ recipe): 260 calories; 12 g protein; 7 g total fat; 3 g saturated fat; 35 g carbohydrates; 3 g fibre; 401 mg sodium

---

* You may make your own breadcrumbs by processing gluten-free, soy-free bread into crumbs in a food processor. Breads that include soy lecithin are suitable on the low-FODMAP diet.

Non-stick cooking spray

225 g gluten-free pasta spirals

400 g peeled and seeded kabocha or other suitable winter squash, cut into 1-cm cubes

60 g dried gluten-free, soy-free breadcrumbs*

60 g grated cheddar

One 425-g tin crushed tomatoes

2 medium courgette grated

5 large eggs, lightly beaten

40 g grated Parmesan

15 g roughly chopped flat-leaf parsley

1 heaped tablespoon ground cumin

1 heaped teaspoon mustard powder

Salt and freshly ground black pepper

Tuna Macaroni and Cheese Bake

SERVES 6–8

Tuna adds a new element to this classic comforting bake, but if you prefer a more traditional macaroni and cheese, you can leave it out. Another play on flavours is to replace the tuna with some tomato passata and cooked chopped bacon or crumbled sautéed tempeh.

1. Bring a large pot of water to a boil. Preheat the oven to 180°C. Grease a 2-litre baking dish with cooking spray.

2. Add the pasta to the boiling water and cook according to packet directions, until just tender. Drain, then return to the pot and cover to keep warm.

3. Combine the breadcrumbs and Parmesan and set aside.

4. Blend 60 ml of the milk with the cornflour in a medium bowl to form a paste. Add the remaining milk, whisking well to remove any lumps. Pour into a saucepan and stir over medium heat until thickened – don't let it boil. Add the cheddar and salt and pepper to taste and stir until melted, then stir in the tuna.

5. Pour the cheese sauce over the pasta and mix until combined. Transfer to the baking dish and top with the Parmesan and breadcrumbs. Bake for 15 to 20 minutes, until bubbling and golden.

PER SERVING (⅛ recipe): 311 calories; 24 g protein; 9 g total fat; 5 g saturated fat; 32 g carbohydrates; 1 g fibre; 609 mg sodium

---

* You may make your own breadcrumbs by processing gluten-free, soy-free bread into crumbs in a food processor. Breads that include soy lecithin are suitable on the low-FODMAP diet.

Non-stick cooking spray

225 g gluten-free macaroni

40 g dried gluten-free, soy-free breadcrumbs*

25 g grated Parmesan

560 ml semi-skimmed milk, lactose-free milk or suitable plant-based milk

50 g cornflour

240 g grated reduced-fat cheddar

Salt and freshly ground black pepper

One 340-g tin tuna packed in water, drained

Lasagna

SERVES 8

Although this recipe suggests using gluten-free lasagna sheets, you could use spring roll wrappers instead. Soak three wrappers together to equal one lasagna sheet. It works really well as an interesting alternative.

1. Preheat the oven to 180°C.

2. Heat the olive oil and the garlic-infused oil in a large heavy-bottomed frying pan over medium heat. Add the beef and bacon and cook until the beef is nicely browned, breaking up any lumps as you go. Spoon off any excess fat, then add the cayenne, chilli powder (if using), tomato passata and carrot. Season with salt and pepper. Simmer over medium heat for 10 minutes, stirring occasionally, until the flavours meld.

3. Blend 60 ml of the milk with the cornflour in a medium bowl to form a paste. Add the remaining milk, whisking well to remove any lumps. Pour into a saucepan and stir over medium heat until thickened – don't let it boil. Add the cheddar and stir until melted. Season to taste with salt and pepper.

4. Prepare the lasagna sheets according to the packet directions. Place a layer of one third of the lasagna sheets over the bottom of a 28 x 18 cm baking pan, breaking them to fit if necessary. Spread half of the meat mixture evenly over the top. Spread one third of the cheese sauce over the meat. Repeat with another layer of lasagna sheets, the remaining meat mixture and half the remaining cheese sauce. Finish with a final layer of lasagna sheets and the rest of the cheese sauce. Bake for 20 minutes or until bubbling and golden. Let sit for a few minutes before cutting.

PER SERVING: 758 calories; 50 g protein; 29 g total fat; 13 g saturated fat; 64 g carbohydrates; 6 g fibre; 1050 mg sodium

2 tablespoons olive oil

2 teaspoons garlic-infused olive oil

900 g extra-lean minced beef

113 g lean bacon slices, diced

2 teaspoons cayenne pepper

½ teaspoon chilli powder (optional)

One 794-g jar tomato passata

1 carrot, grated

Salt and freshly ground black pepper

1 litre skimmed milk, lactose-free milk or suitable plant-based milk

3 tablespoons cornflour

360 g grated reduced-fat cheddar

450 g gluten-free lasagna sheets

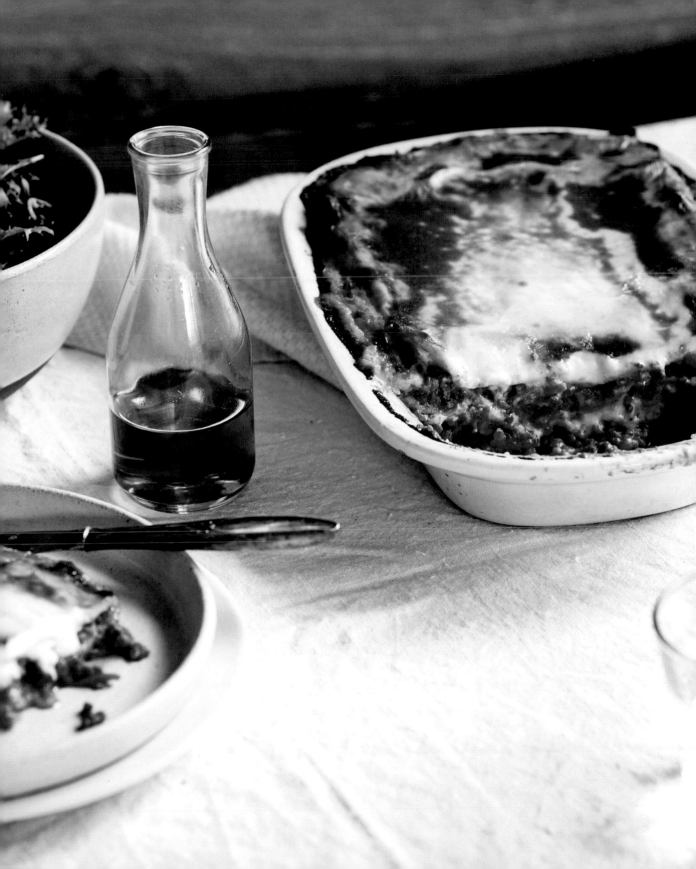

Smoked Tuna Risotto

SERVES 6

Smoked food often becomes the flavour highlight of any dish in which it is used. Smoked tuna is no exception, giving an earthy depth to this delicious risotto. If you cannot locate it, however, a 340-g tin of regular tuna also suits this risotto (ideally with the addition of ¼ teaspoon of cayenne pepper and 115 g of diced roasted red peppers). With the tuna and/or Parmesan left out or replaced with tofu, this dish is also an excellent option for vegetarians or vegans, especially with a handful of crushed toasted walnuts as a garnish.

1. Pour the stock into a medium saucepan. Cover and bring to a gentle simmer over low heat.

2. Meanwhile, heat the olive oil and garlic-infused oil in a large heavy-bottomed saucepan over medium heat. Add the saffron and cook, stirring, for 2 minutes. Add the rice and stir until it is well coated in the oil and saffron.

3. Add the wine to the rice and cook until absorbed. Add 250 ml of the hot stock and cook, stirring, until it is completely absorbed. Repeat this process, adding 125 ml stock at a time, until just 125 ml of the stock remains.

4. Add the tuna, peas, courgette, Parmesan and parsley and stir until well combined. Pour in the remaining stock and stir until the stock is nearly absorbed and the rice is tender. Season to taste with salt and pepper and serve.

PER SERVING: 548 calories; 28 g protein; 8 g total fat; 1 g saturated fat; 82 g carbohydrates; 4 g fibre; 926 mg sodium

---

* Most stocks contain onion or garlic. Choose one that is onion-free. If garlic is present, the amount is likely to be minimal and should be suitable for most people on a low-FODMAP diet. If you are extremely sensitive to garlic, omit the stock and use water instead, or make your own stock by boiling chicken bones and/or suitable vegetables (including carrot and celery) in water with your choice of seasonings for about an hour, then straining out the solids.

2 litres gluten-free, onion-free chicken or vegetable stock*

2 teaspoons olive oil

2 teaspoons garlic-infused olive oil

2 saffron threads

500 g Arborio rice

125 ml white wine

385 g tinned or packaged smoked tuna, drained and flaked

120 g frozen peas

2 medium courgettes, halved lengthwise and sliced

40 g grated Parmesan

15 g roughly chopped flat-leaf parsley

Salt and freshly ground black pepper

Beef Risotto with Whole Grain Mustard and Spinach

SERVES 6

Mustard is a natural partner for steak or roast beef, so I just knew they would taste great together as the base flavours for this risotto.

1. Heat the garlic-infused oil in a large frying pan over medium heat and cook the beef, stirring occasionally, until lightly browned. Add the spinach and cook until wilted. Set aside.

2. Pour the stock into a medium saucepan. Cover and bring to a gentle simmer over low heat.

3. Heat the olive oil in a large heavy-bottomed saucepan over medium heat. Add the rice and stir until it is well coated in the oil. Add 125 ml of the hot stock and cook, stirring, until the stock has been completely absorbed. Repeat this process, adding 125 ml of the stock at a time, until just 125 ml stock remains. Stir in the beef and spinach, the Parmesan, mustard and chopped parsley. Add the remaining stock and cook, stirring, until it is nearly absorbed and the rice is tender. Spoon into six bowls and garnish with the parsley sprigs.

PER SERVING: 624 calories; 25 g protein; 20 g total fat; 5 g saturated fat; 83 g carbohydrates; 3 g fibre; 869 mg sodium

---

* Most stocks contain onion or garlic. Choose one that is onion-free. If garlic is present, the amount is likely to be minimal and should be suitable for most people on a low-FODMAP diet. If you are extremely sensitive to garlic, omit the stock and use water instead, or make your own stock by boiling beef bones and/or suitable vegetables (including carrot and celery) in water with your choice of seasonings for about an hour, then straining out the solids.

2 teaspoons garlic-infused olive oil

450 g lean beef, cut into strips

225 g baby spinach leaves, rinsed and dried

2 litres gluten-free, onion-free beef stock*

2 teaspoons olive oil

500 g Arborio rice

60 g grated Parmesan

95 g gluten-free wholegrain mustard

2 heaped tablespoons roughly chopped flat-leaf parsley, plus sprigs for garnish

Asian Duck and Pea Risotto

SERVES 8

Duck can be purchased from Asian markets and certain super-markets and adds flavours that complement Asian ingredients well. If you can't find duck, use chicken instead.

1. Cut the flesh from 2 of the duck quarters into 2-cm strips. Discard the skin and bones.

2. Combine the soy sauce, garlic-infused oil, ginger and 1 tablespoon of the sesame oil in a large bowl. Season with salt and pepper. Add the duck strips and the remaining quarters and toss to coat. Cover and refrigerate for 3 to 4 hours or overnight.

3. Preheat the oven to 180°C. Pour the stock into a medium saucepan. Cover and bring to a gentle simmer over low heat.

4. Reserving the strips and marinade, place the duck quarters in a baking dish. Roast for 25 to 30 minutes, until cooked through (liquid should run clear when a thigh is pierced with a toothpick in the thickest part). Cover loosely with foil and keep warm.

5. While the duck quarters are roasting, heat the remaining 1 tablespoon sesame oil in a large heavy-bottomed saucepan over medium heat, add the celery and cook until tender and slightly browned. Add the rice and stir until it is well coated in the oil and celery. Add the duck strips and any remaining marinade.

6. Add 125 ml of the hot stock and cook, stirring, until it has been completely absorbed. Repeat this process, adding 125 ml of the stock at a time, until the rice is tender. Add the peas with the last of the stock, cook until the stock is nearly absorbed and the peas are thawed and warmed through. Season with salt and pepper to taste. Spoon the risotto onto six plates and top each with a roasted duck quarter and another grinding of pepper.

PER SERVING: 536 calories; 32 g protein; 15 g total fat; 3 g saturated fat; 61 g carbohydrates; 2 g fibre; 1434 mg sodium

Eight 170-g duck leg quarters (leg and thigh)

125 ml gluten-free soy sauce

2 teaspoons garlic-infused olive oil

2 teaspoons grated ginger

2 tablespoons sesame oil

Salt and freshly ground black pepper

2 litres gluten-free, onion-free chicken stock*

2 celery stalks, sliced

500 g Arborio rice

120 g frozen peas

---

* Most stocks contain onion or garlic. Choose one that is onion-free. If garlic is present, the amount is likely to be minimal and should be suitable for most people on a low-FODMAP diet. If you are extremely sensitive to garlic, omit the stock and use water instead, or make your own stock by boiling chicken bones and/or suitable vegetables (including carrot and celery) in water with your choice of seasonings for about an hour, then straining out the solids.

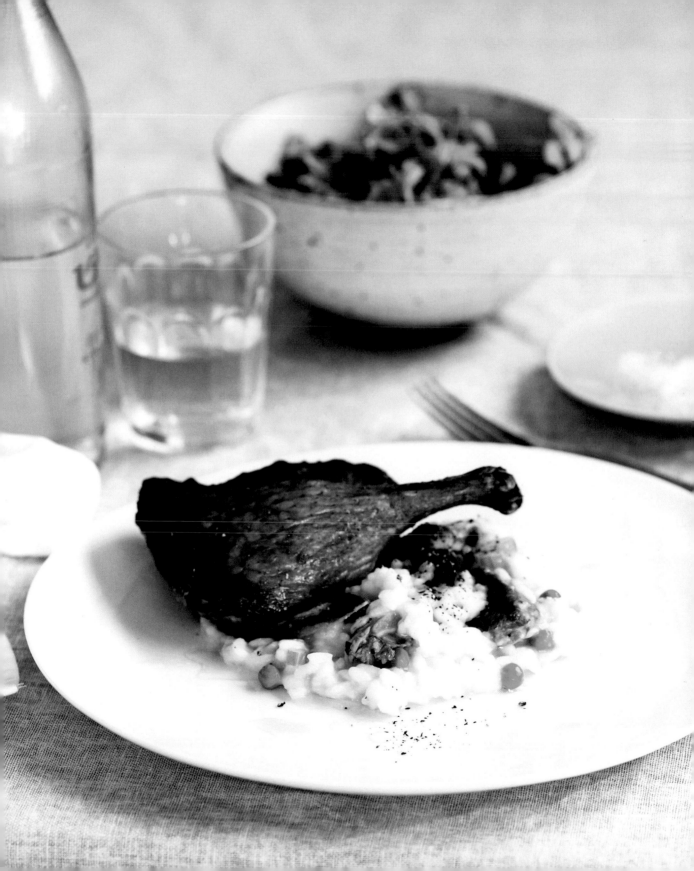

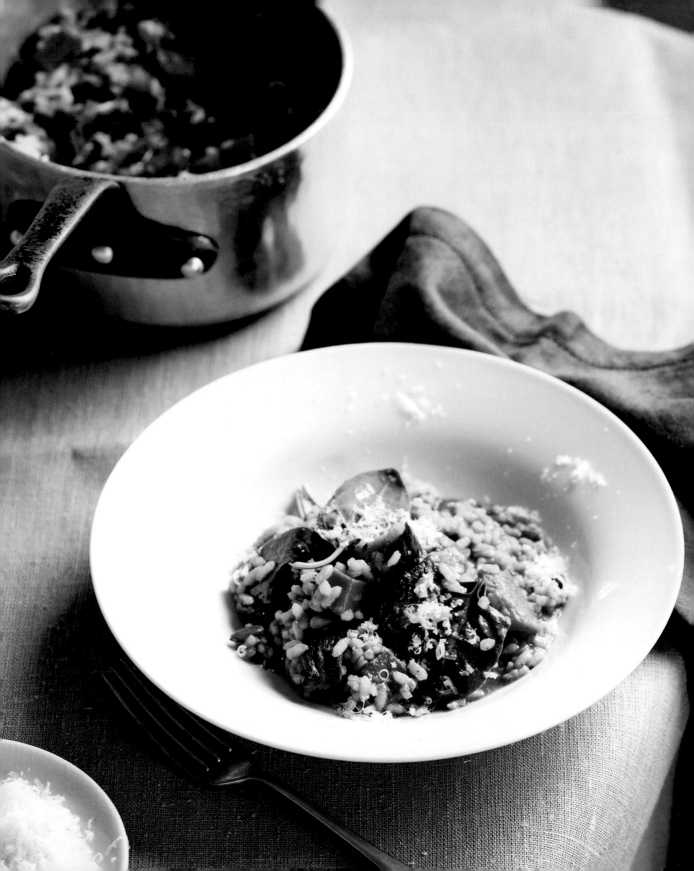

Lamb and Aubergine Risotto with Middle Eastern Spices

SERVES 6

I don't remember eating aubergine when I was a child, and what a shame! I have certainly embraced it now, and enjoy cooking it in many ways, including this Middle Eastern–inspired risotto.

1. Preheat the oven to 180°C.

2. Spread the squash on one baking sheet and the aubergine on another. Brush them both with garlic-infused oil and bake for 20 to 30 minutes, until tender and just beginning to go brown. Set the squash aside to cool, and wrap the aubergine in foil to sweat for 10 minutes. Remove the aubergine from the foil and roughly chop. Set aside.

3. Heat 1 tablespoon garlic-infused oil in a large heavy-bottomed saucepan over medium heat. Add the cumin, coriander, turmeric, cardamom and sumac and cook until fragrant. Add the lamb strips and toss to coat in the spices. Cook the lamb, stirring occasionally, until just cooked through. Transfer the lamb to a bowl and set aside. Do not wash the saucepan.

4. Pour the stock into a medium saucepan. Cover and bring to a gentle simmer over low heat.

5. Add the rice to the pan you cooked the meat in and cook over medium heat, stirring, for 2 to 3 minutes. Add 250 ml of the stock and cook, stirring, until nearly all the stock has been absorbed. Repeat this process, adding 125 ml of stock at a time, until just 125 ml stock remains.

6. Stir in the lamb, squash, aubergine, pine nuts, Parmesan and spinach. Add the remaining stock and cook, stirring, until the stock is nearly absorbed and the rice is tender. Spoon into 6 bowls and serve with an extra sprinkling of Parmesan, if desired.

PER SERVING (not including optional Parmesan for serving): 654 calories; 26 g protein; 20 g total fat; 6 g saturated fat; 87 g carbohydrates; 4 g fibre; 778 mg sodium

300 g peeled and seeded kabocha or other suitable winter squash, cut into 2-cm cubes

1 medium-small (100 g) aubergine

Garlic-infused olive oil

1½ teaspoons ground cumin

1 teaspoon ground coriander

1 teaspoon ground turmeric

¼ teaspoon ground cardamom

¼ teaspoon ground sumac, or ¼ teaspoon paprika plus ½ teaspoon grated lemon zest

450 g lean lamb, cut into strips

2.5 litres gluten-free, onion-free beef stock*

500 g Arborio rice

50 g pine nuts, toasted

40 g grated Parmesan, plus more for serving (optional)

2 handfuls of baby spinach leaves, rinsed and dried

---

* Choose a stock that is onion-free. If garlic is present, the amount is likely to be minimal and should be suitable for most people on a low-FODMAP diet. If you are extremely sensitive to garlic, use water instead, or make your own stock by boiling chicken bones and/or suitable vegetables (including carrot and celery) in water with your choice of seasonings for about an hour, then straining out the solids.

Grilled Snapper on Lemon and Spinach Risotto

SERVES 4

This dish was inspired by a fabulous dinner I had in a restaurant on a lovely warm summer's evening in Northern Australia many years ago. You can add more lemon zest if you like a more intense citrus flavour.

1. To make the risotto, pour the stock into a medium saucepan. Cover and bring to a gentle simmer over low heat.

2. Heat the olive oil, garlic-infused oil, lemon juice and zest in a large heavy-bottomed saucepan over medium heat. Add the rice and stir until it is well coated.

3. Add 250 ml of the hot stock and cook, stirring, until it has been completely absorbed. Repeat this process, adding 125 ml of the stock at a time, until just 125 ml stock remains. Stir in the spinach, Parmesan and parsley. Add the remaining stock and cook, stirring, until it is nearly absorbed and the rice is tender. Season to taste with salt and pepper. Cover and keep warm.

4. When you add the spinach to the risotto, preheat the grill to high.

5. Dust the snapper fillets in cornflour. Grill for 4 to 6 minutes, until crispy. Turn and grill the other side until just cooked through.

6. Serve the snapper with the risotto and a fresh green salad.

PER SERVING (not including the green salad): 342 calories; 16 g protein; 12 g total fat; 1 g saturated fat; 41 g carbohydrates; 1 g fibre; 658 mg sodium

* Most stocks contain onion or garlic. Choose one that is onion-free. If garlic is present, the amount is likely to be minimal and should be suitable for most people on a low-FODMAP diet. If you are extremely sensitive to garlic, omit the stock and use water instead, or make your own stock by boiling chicken bones and/or suitable vegetables (including carrot and celery) in water with your choice of seasonings for about an hour, then straining out the solids.

LEMON AND SPINACH RISOTTO

1 litre gluten-free, onion-free chicken or vegetable stock*

2 tablespoons olive oil

2 teaspoons garlic-infused olive oil

80 ml fresh lemon juice

1 heaped tablespoon finely grated lemon zest

130 g Arborio rice

Handful of baby spinach leaves, rinsed and dried

25 g grated Parmesan

2 heaped tablespoons finely chopped flat-leaf parsley

Salt and freshly ground black pepper

Four 200-g snapper or barramundi fillets

35 g cornflour

Green salad, for serving

Chicken Risotto with Roasted Squash and Sage

SERVES 6

Sage is a classic, versatile herb that goes particularly well with squash, but you could also use chives, oregano or rosemary in this dish if you prefer them.

1. Preheat the oven to 200°C.

2. Spread the squash on a baking sheet and brush with a little of the olive oil. Bake for 30 minutes, or until soft and browned. Remove from the oven and select 4 perfect pieces for the garnish.

3. Pour the stock into a medium saucepan. Cover and bring to a gentle simmer over low heat.

4. Heat the remaining olive oil and the garlic-infused oil in a large heavy-bottomed saucepan over medium heat. Add the chicken and sage and cook, stirring, for 2 minutes. Add the rice and stir until it is well coated in the oil and sage.

5. Add 250 ml of the hot stock and the squash (except the pieces for garnish) and cook, stirring, until the stock has been completely absorbed. Repeat this process, adding 125 ml of the stock at a time, until the rice is tender. Add the Parmesan and parsley and stir until just combined and the cheese is starting to melt. Season to taste with salt and pepper and serve garnished with the reserved squash pieces.

PER SERVING: 485 calories; 22 g protein; 9 g total fat; 1 g saturated fat; 75 g carbohydrates; 3 g fibre; 647 mg sodium

One 1 kg kabocha or other suitable winter squash, peeled, seeded and cut into 2-cm cubes

2 tablespoons olive oil

1.5 litres gluten-free, onion-free chicken or vegetable stock*

2 teaspoons garlic-infused olive oil

340 g boneless, skinless chicken breasts, diced

12 sage leaves, roughly chopped

400 g Arborio rice

40 g grated Parmesan

2 heaped tablespoons roughly chopped flat-leaf parsley

Salt and freshly ground black pepper

---

* Most stocks contain onion or garlic. Choose one that is onion-free. If garlic is present, the amount is likely to be minimal and should be suitable for most people on a low-FODMAP diet. If you are extremely sensitive to garlic, omit the stock and use water instead, or make your own stock by boiling chicken bones and/or suitable vegetables (including carrot and celery) in water with your choice of seasonings for about an hour, then straining out the solids.

Chicken Fried Rice

SERVES 4

This recipe is more complex than regular fried rice. The sliced chicken and aromatic spices make it warmly comforting and satisfying. Those who don't eat chicken can enjoy this recipe using thinly sliced well-pressed tofu, and the eggs can be left out if necessary. A sprinkling of crushed low-FODMAP nuts would be a nice touch.

1. Cook the rice following packet instructions until just tender. Drain well and chill, preferably for several hours or overnight.

2. Heat the garlic-infused oil and olive oil in a large frying pan or wok over medium heat. Add the five-spice powder, cumin and ginger and cook until fragrant. Add the chicken and stir-fry until just cooked through, 4 to 5 minutes.

3. Add the carrot, peas, red pepper, bamboo shoots and bean sprouts and toss to combine. Make a well in the middle, add the eggs and stir until the eggs are just cooked, breaking up the eggs as you go. Cook until the pepper and carrot are tender, then add the rice and toss to combine.

4. Just before serving, stir in the soy sauce and sesame oil. Sprinkle the coriander leaves on top and serve immediately.

PER SERVING: 625 calories; 40 g protein; 13 g total fat; 3 g saturated fat; 84 g carbohydrates; 4 g fibre; 1051 mg sodium

400 g white or brown long-grain rice

2 teaspoons garlic-infused olive oil

2 teaspoons olive oil

1½ teaspoons Chinese five-spice powder

½ teaspoon ground cumin

1 heaped tablespoon grated ginger

450 g boneless, skinless chicken breasts, thinly sliced

1 large carrot, cut into matchsticks

60 g fresh or frozen peas

½ red pepper, seeded and cut into matchsticks

One 225-g tin bamboo shoots, drained

80 g bean sprouts

2 large eggs, lightly beaten

60 ml gluten-free soy sauce

1 tablespoon toasted sesame oil

Coriander leaves, to garnish

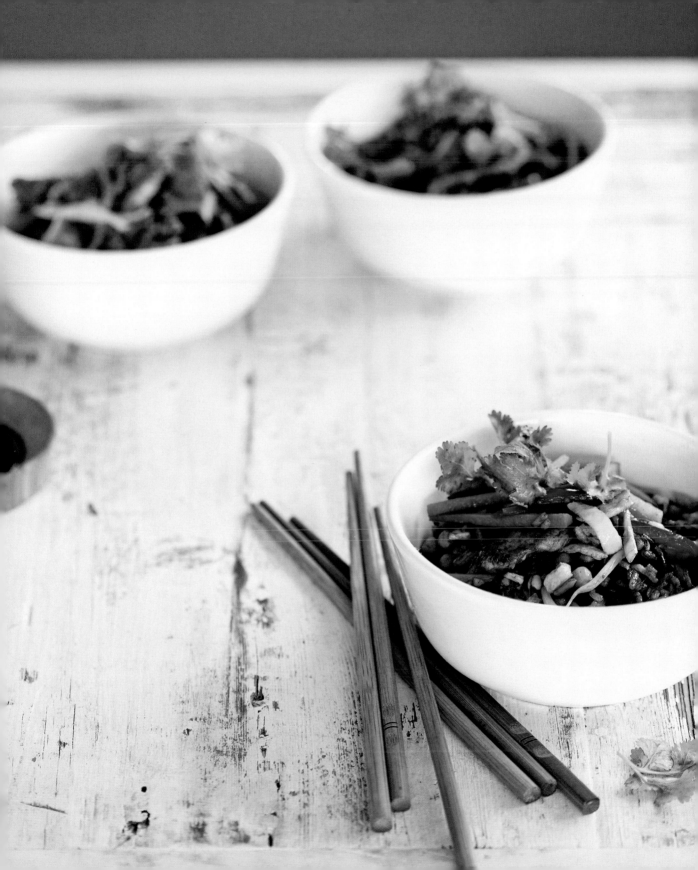

PIZZA

SERVES 4

It is so easy to make a fresh pizza crust, but if you are pressed for time, ready-made gluten-free pizza crusts are available from the health food section of larger supermarkets, or you can use gluten-free pita bread. I've given a couple of topping suggestions here but the beauty of pizza is that you can use whatever you like.

Pizza Crust

280 g gluten-free, soy-free bread or pizza mix
2 teaspoons olive oil

1. Preheat the oven to 120°C, or follow the packet directions. Line a pizza stone or baking sheet with parchment paper.
2. Make the gluten-free bread mix following the packet directions, then spoon it onto the parchment paper. Using the back of a metal spoon, dipped in water if needed, spread the dough into a large circle (about 30 cm in diameter). Brush the pizza crust with the olive oil and bake for 15 minutes, or until lightly browned.
3. Increase the oven temperature to 180°C. Top the crust with your choice of ingredients and cook for 15 minutes, or until the toppings are warmed through and the cheese (if using) has melted.

PER SERVING: 245 calories; 8 g protein; 2 g total fat; 0 g saturated fat; 3 g carbohydrates; 5 g fibre; mg sodium

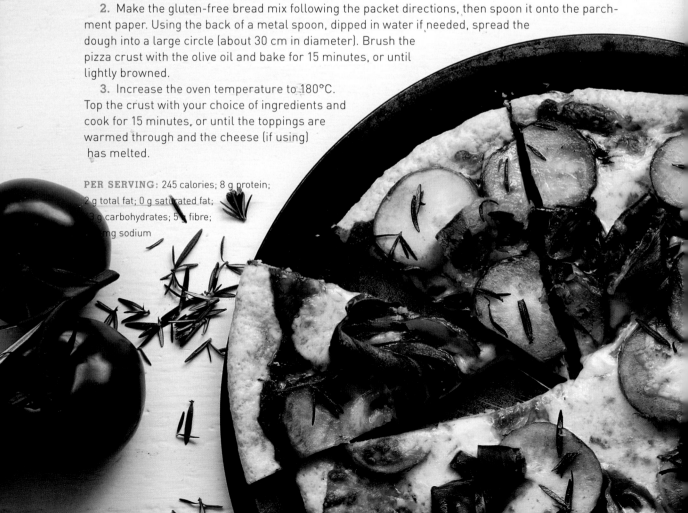

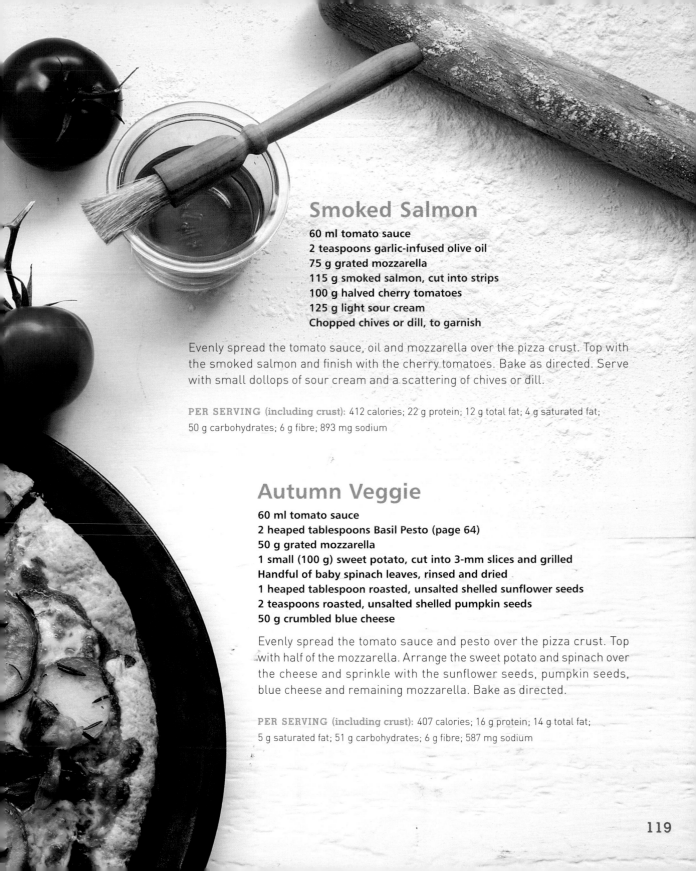

Smoked Salmon

60 ml tomato sauce
2 teaspoons garlic-infused olive oil
75 g grated mozzarella
115 g smoked salmon, cut into strips
100 g halved cherry tomatoes
125 g light sour cream
Chopped chives or dill, to garnish

Evenly spread the tomato sauce, oil and mozzarella over the pizza crust. Top with the smoked salmon and finish with the cherry tomatoes. Bake as directed. Serve with small dollops of sour cream and a scattering of chives or dill.

PER SERVING (including crust): 412 calories; 22 g protein; 12 g total fat; 4 g saturated fat; 50 g carbohydrates; 6 g fibre; 893 mg sodium

Autumn Veggie

60 ml tomato sauce
2 heaped tablespoons Basil Pesto (page 64)
50 g grated mozzarella
1 small (100 g) sweet potato, cut into 3-mm slices and grilled
Handful of baby spinach leaves, rinsed and dried
1 heaped tablespoon roasted, unsalted shelled sunflower seeds
2 teaspoons roasted, unsalted shelled pumpkin seeds
50 g crumbled blue cheese

Evenly spread the tomato sauce and pesto over the pizza crust. Top with half of the mozzarella. Arrange the sweet potato and spinach over the cheese and sprinkle with the sunflower seeds, pumpkin seeds, blue cheese and remaining mozzarella. Bake as directed.

PER SERVING (including crust): 407 calories; 16 g protein; 14 g total fat; 5 g saturated fat; 51 g carbohydrates; 6 g fibre; 587 mg sodium

Pesto Margherita

2 heaped tablespoons Basil Pesto (page 64)
50 g grated mozzarella
3 to 4 mozzarella bocconcini, thinly sliced
2 medium tomatoes, sliced
Torn basil leaves, to garnish

Evenly spread the pesto over the pizza crust and top with the grated mozzarella. Add a layer of bocconcini and a layer of tomatoes. Bake as directed. Serve garnished with the basil leaves.

PER SERVING (including crust): 396 calories; 17 g protein; 14 g total fat; 5 g saturated fat; 46 g carbohydrates; 6 g fibre; 338 mg sodium

Potato and Rosemary

2 small red-skin potatoes, peeled (if desired)
2 teaspoons garlic-infused olive oil
2 teaspoons olive oil
2 heaped tablespoons roughly chopped rosemary
60 ml tomato sauce
50 g grated mozzarella (optional)
40 g roughly chopped thinly sliced prosciutto, or 35 g roughly chopped grilled courgette or aubergine

1. Place the whole potatoes in a medium saucepan and cover with cold water. Bring to a boil over high heat, then reduce the heat to medium-high and boil for 10 to 12 minutes, until just tender. Drain. Allow to cool slightly, then slice as thinly as possible.

2. Heat the garlic-infused oil and olive oil in a large frying pan, add the potato slices and rosemary, and cook until the potatoes are golden brown on both sides.

3. Evenly spread the tomato sauce over the pizza crust and scatter the mozzarella across the top, if using. Arrange the potatoes and prosciutto on top. Bake as directed.

PER SERVING (including crust; with prosciutto): 379 calories; 15 g protein; 12 g total fat; 3 g saturated fat; 48 g carbohydrates; 7 g fibre; 645 mg sodium

Grilled Fish with Coconut-Lime Rice

SERVES 4

This little recipe is so easy to make but gives a massive hit of flavour. The chilli pepper gives a good heat to the fish, but you can leave it out if you prefer. It will still taste great.

1. Place all the ingredients for the marinade in a large glass or ceramic bowl and stir to combine well. Add the fish fillets and toss gently to coat. Cover and place in the refrigerator for 2 to 3 hours, turning every hour to ensure even marinating.

2. Bring a large pot of water to a boil over high heat. Reduce the heat to medium, add the rice and one third of the lime leaves, and cook, stirring occasionally, for 10 minutes, or until the rice is tender. Drain and rinse under hot water.

3. Place the rinsed rice in a bowl and stir in the coconut milk and remaining lime leaves. Cover and keep warm.

4. Brush a ridged grill pan or cast-iron frying pan with the garlic-infused oil and heat over medium-high heat. Drain the fish fillets and cook for 2 to 3 minutes on each side, until cooked to your preferred doneness.

5. Serve with the coconut-lime rice.

PER SERVING: 475 calories; 33 g protein; 11g total fat; 6 g saturated fat; 59 g carbohydrates; 2 g fibre; 92 mg sodium

MARINADE

1 tablespoon plus 1 teaspoon fresh lemon juice

1 tablespoon plus 1 teaspoon sesame oil

1 teaspoon garlic-infused olive oil

¼ small red chilli, seeded and finely chopped (optional)

Freshly ground black pepper

4 large boneless, skinless firm white fish fillets (such as snapper or cod; 160 g each)

300 g jasmine rice

3 kaffir lime leaves, very thinly sliced

125 ml coconut milk

Garlic-infused olive oil

Baked Atlantic Salmon on Soft Blue Cheese Polenta

SERVES 4

If you haven't cooked polenta before, this is the dish to try. I have so many requests for it when I entertain, which is fine with me as it is super easy! If you're not a fan of blue cheese, just use Parmesan instead. The garlic is used only to infuse the milk with flavour and should be well tolerated; be sure to remember to remove it, though.

1. Preheat the oven to 180°C. Brush a baking sheet lightly with olive oil.

2. Place the salmon fillets on the baking sheet, brush with olive oil and bake for 10 to 12 minutes, until cooked to your preferred doneness.

3. Meanwhile, combine the milk and garlic in a medium saucepan over medium heat and bring to just below a boil. Remove the garlic with a slotted spoon and discard. Add the cornmeal to the milk and stir until the polenta comes to a boil. Reduce the heat to low and cook, stirring constantly, for 3 to 5 minutes more. The polenta should be the texture of smooth mashed potatoes. Stir in the blue cheese and allow to melt. Season to taste with salt and pepper.

4. Spoon the polenta onto warmed plates, top with the salmon fillets, and serve with your choice of salad or vegetables.

PER SERVING (not including the green salad): 556 calories; 44 g protein; 29 g total fat; 9 g saturated fat; 27 g carbohydrates; 2 g fibre; 490 mg sodium

Olive oil

Four 160-g Atlantic salmon fillets, skin on, pin bones removed

750 ml semi-skimmed milk, lactose-free milk or suitable plant-based milk

2 garlic cloves, peeled and halved

110 g coarse cornmeal (instant polenta)

90 g strong blue cheese (or to taste)

Salt and freshly ground black pepper

Green salad or vegetables, for serving

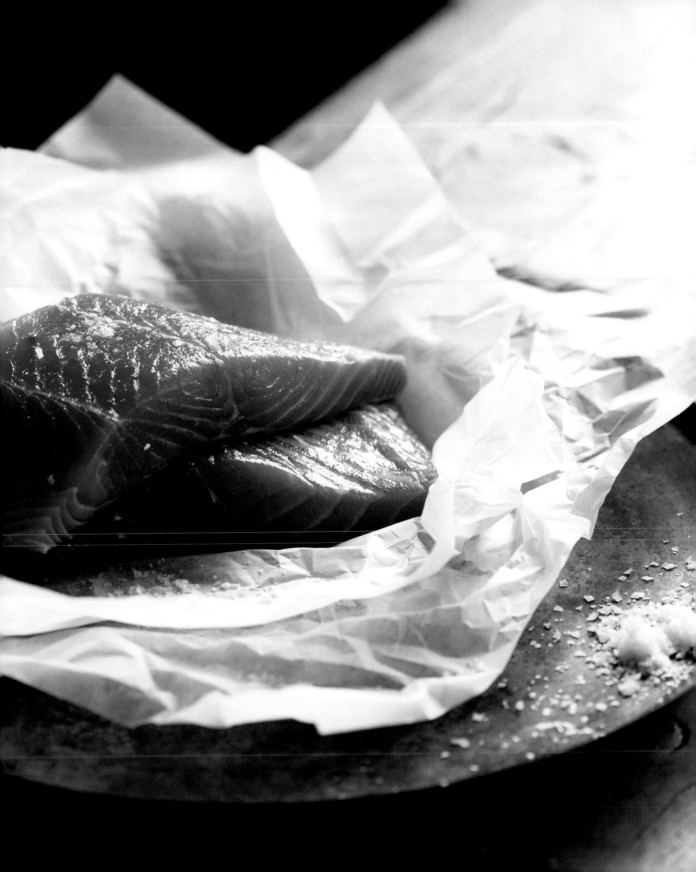

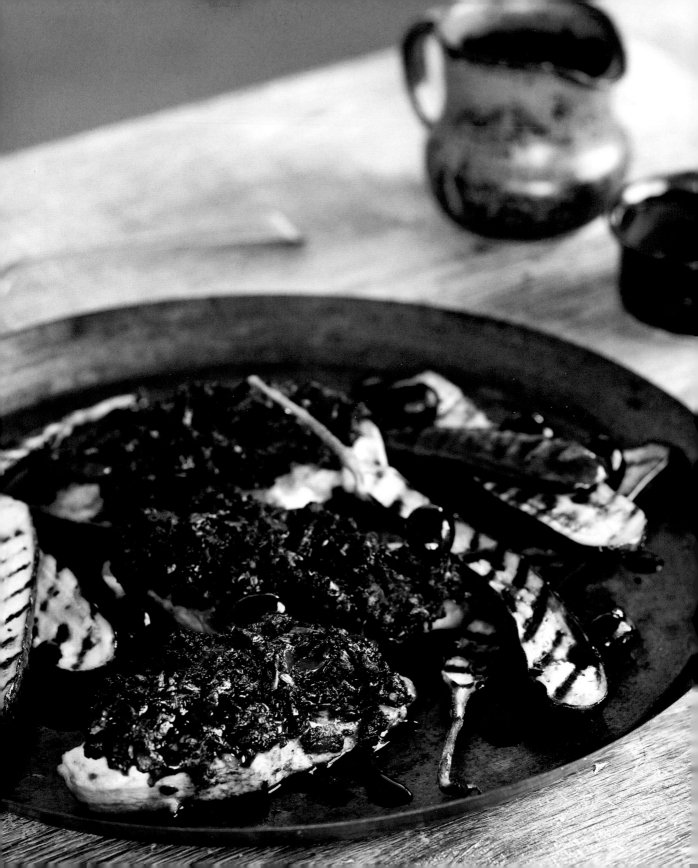

Chicken with Olives, Sun-Dried Tomato and Basil with Mediterranean Vegetables

SERVES 4

Classic flavours of the Mediterranean make this a winning dish. Double the quantities if you are feeding a crowd.

1. Preheat the oven to 170°C. Line a baking sheet with parchment paper.

2. Using a mortar and pestle, crush the black olives, sun-dried tomatoes, basil, 1 tablespoon of the olive oil and salt and pepper to taste into an even paste (it can be as smooth or chunky as you like). If you don't have a mortar and pestle, use a blender or mini food processor.

3. Heat the remaining 1 tablespoon of olive oil in a large frying pan over medium-low heat. Add the chicken breasts and pan-fry for 5 minutes on each side, until lightly browned and cooked through.

4. Transfer the chicken to the prepared baking sheet and spoon the olive paste over the top. Cover with foil and bake for 10 to 15 minutes.

5. Meanwhile, to make the Mediterranean vegetables, spray a ridged grill pan or cast-iron frying pan with cooking spray and heat over medium heat. Add the courgette and aubergine (in batches, if necessary) and cook for 3 to 4 minutes on each side, until tender. Add the kalamata olives and warm through.

6. Lightly drizzle both the chicken and the vegetables with balsamic vinegar and serve together.

PER SERVING: 363 calories; 41 g protein; 16 g total fat; 2 g saturated fat; 13 g carbohydrates; 4 g fibre; 505 mg sodium

2 heaped tablespoons pitted black or kalamata olives

75 g sun-dried tomatoes, drained (if packed in oil)

Small handful of basil leaves

2 tablespoons olive oil

Salt and freshly ground black pepper

Four 170-g boneless, skinless chicken breasts

MEDITERRANEAN VEGETABLES

Non-stick cooking spray

2 small courgettes, thinly sliced lengthwise

1 small (80 g) aubergine, thinly sliced lengthwise

80 g kalamata olives, pitted

2 tablespoons plus 2 teaspoons balsamic vinegar

Spanish Chicken with Creamy Herbed Rice

SERVES 4

During summer I love to serve this cold for Sunday lunch. But you can also enjoy it warm – simply use warm rice and serve the chicken straight from the pan.

1. Preheat the oven to 180°C.

2. Combine the garlic-infused oil, paprika, cumin, turmeric, salt and pepper in a small bowl. Place the chicken in a large baking dish and rub with about three quarters of the spice mixture.

3. Bake the chicken for 20 minutes or until cooked through. Remove from the oven, reserve any cooking juices separately and set aside for 1 to 2 hours.

4. To make the creamy herbed rice, combine all the ingredients in a large bowl and mix together well.

5. Combine the remaining spice mix and the cooking juices with a little water in a small frying pan over medium heat. Simmer until warmed through.

6. Cut the chicken into thick slices and serve at room temperature with the rice, a drizzle of the spicy sauce and a scattering of mint or parsley leaves. Serve cold or at room temperature.

PER SERVING: 593 calories; 47 g protein; 35 g total fat; 6 g saturated fat; 37 g carbohydrates; 2 g fibre; 385 mg sodium

2 tablespoons plus 2 teaspoons garlic-infused olive oil

1 heaped tablespoon smoked paprika

1 heaped tablespoon ground cumin

½ teaspoon ground turmeric

Salt and freshly ground black pepper

Four 170-g boneless, skinless chicken breasts

CREAMY HERBED RICE

300 g cooked basmati rice, at room temperature (made from 130 g uncooked rice)

2 teaspoons garlic-infused olive oil

3 tablespoons olive oil

60 ml red wine vinegar

200 g gluten-free low-fat plain yogurt

90 g Basil Pesto (page 64)

15 g flat-leaf parsley leaves

2 heaped tablespoons finely chopped mint

Mint or flat-leaf parsley leaves, for garnish

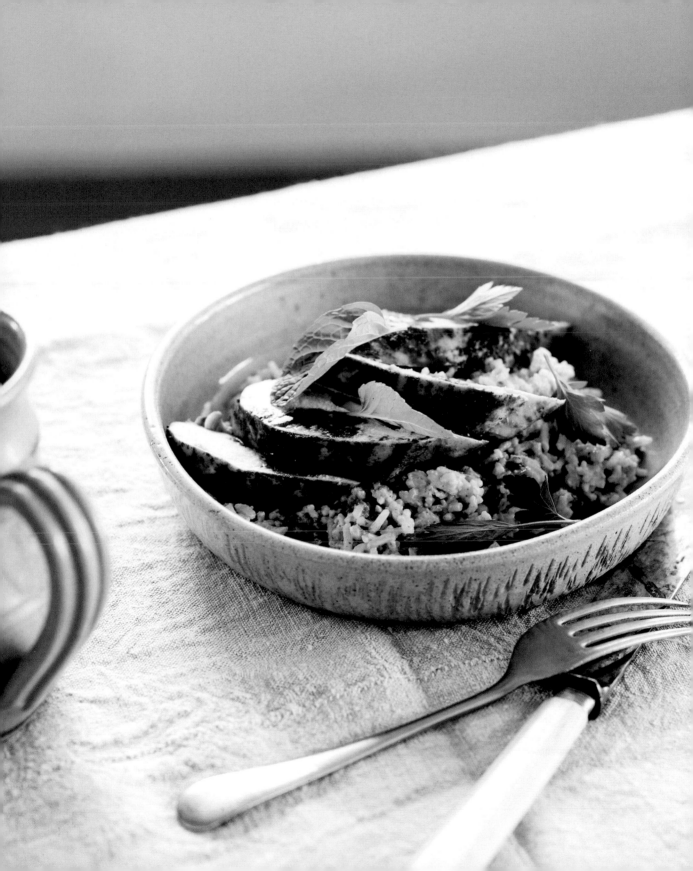

Chicken and Vegetable Curry

SERVES 4

This is an Indian-style curry, but it's not laden with onion (high in FODMAPs) or ghee (high in fat). It is just lightly spiced with plenty of chicken and vegetables, so even kids and picky eaters should enjoy it.

1. Heat the garlic-infused oil and olive oil in a large heavy-bottomed saucepan or Dutch oven over medium heat. Add the garam masala, cumin, turmeric, cayenne and sesame oil, and cook for 1 to 2 minutes, until fragrant.

2. Add the chicken, tomatoes, courgette, green beans, squash, brown sugar and 125 ml water. Reduce the heat to medium-low, then cover and cook, stirring occasionally, until the chicken and vegetables are tender and the sauce has thickened.

3. Serve with steamed rice.

PER SERVING (not including the rice): 496 calories; 43 g protein; 21 g total fat; 4 g saturated fat; 32 g carbohydrates; 6 g fibre; 193 mg sodium

2 teaspoons garlic-infused olive oil

2 tablespoons olive oil

1 heaped tablespoon garam masala

1 heaped tablespoon ground cumin

2 teaspoons ground turmeric

½ teaspoon cayenne pepper (or to taste)

1 tablespoon sesame oil

Four 200-g boneless, skinless chicken thighs, trimmed of fat

3 Roma (plum) tomatoes, chopped

1 courgette, halved lengthwise and sliced

180 g trimmed and halved green beans

250 g kabocha or other suitable winter squash, peeled, seeded, and cut into 2-cm pieces

55 g light brown sugar

Steamed rice, for serving

Chicken Parmigiana

SERVES 4

There are all sorts of variations on this iconic dish. Because this is a gluten-free, low-FODMAP cookbook there is no onion in the sauce, but don't despair – it still tastes great.

1. Preheat the oven to 180°C.
2. To make the sauce, combine the tomatoes, parsley, paprika, sugar and olives in a small frying pan and cook over medium-low heat for 15 minutes, stirring occasionally.
3. Set out three shallow bowls and fill one with the cornflour, one with the eggs and one with the breadcrumbs mixed with the salt and pepper. Beat the eggs lightly. Coat the chicken breasts in the cornflour, shaking off any excess, then dip in the egg and finally toss in the breadcrumbs until well coated.
4. Heat the olive oil in a large frying pan over medium-low heat. Add the chicken and cook for 3 to 4 minutes on each side, until golden brown and cooked through.
5. Place the chicken breasts in a baking dish, spoon the sauce over them, and top with the cheddar. Cover and bake for 15 minutes, or until the cheese is golden and melted.
6. Serve with your choice of salad or vegetables.

PER SERVING (not including the green salad): 516 calories; 50 g protein; 16 g total fat; 5 g saturated fat; 37 g carbohydrates; 2 g fibre; 805 mg sodium

---

* You may make your own breadcrumbs by processing gluten-free, soy-free bread into crumbs in a food processor. Breads that include soy lecithin are suitable on the low-FODMAP diet.

TOMATO SAUCE

One 425-g tin crushed tomatoes

2 heaped tablespoons chopped flat-leaf parsley

1 teaspoon sweet paprika

2 teaspoons sugar

80 g sliced black olives

75 g cornflour

2 large eggs

120 g dried gluten-free, soy-free breadcrumbs*

Salt and freshly ground black pepper

Four 170-g boneless, skinless chicken breasts

1 tablespoon olive oil

80 g grated reduced-fat Parmesan or cheddar

Green salad or vegetables, for serving

Baked Chicken and Mozzarella Croquettes

SERVES 4

Although there are a few steps to this dish, they are not difficult, and the result is an elegant, flavour-packed meal to serve your friends and family. On special occasions, wrap the croquettes in prosciutto to push the decadence over the top.

1. Preheat the oven to 180°C. Grease a baking sheet with non-stick cooking spray.

2. Combine the chicken, breadcrumbs, egg and pesto in a food processor or blender and process until just combined – do not purée. Divide the mixture into 8 portions and form into balls. Gently flatten each ball and place a piece of mozzarella and a basil leaf in the middle of each. Re-form the balls to enclose the cheese and basil, then shape into croquettes about 5 cm long and 3 cm wide. If using the prosciutto, wrap each croquette in a slice and secure with a toothpick.

3. Place the croquettes on the baking sheet. Bake for 20 minutes, or until the chicken is cooked through (and the prosciutto, if using, is crisp). Test by cutting into a croquette; it should be opaque.

4. Meanwhile, to make the sauce, combine the cream and garlic-infused oil in a small saucepan over medium-low heat and season well with salt and pepper. Cook, stirring, until warmed through.

5. Serve two chicken croquettes per person with the sauce and your choice of salad or vegetables.

PER SERVING (with prosciutto; not including the green salad): 435 calories; 36 g protein; 27 g total fat; 7 g saturated fat; 10 g carbohydrates; 0 g fibre; 899 mg sodium

Non-stick cooking spray

5 large boneless, skinless chicken thighs, excess fat removed, cut into chunks

80 g dried gluten-free, soy-free breadcrumbs*

1 large egg

60 ml Basil Pesto (page 64)

115 g mozzarella, cut into 8 cubes

8 basil leaves

8 prosciutto slices (optional)

GARLIC-INFUSED CREAM SAUCE

60 ml single cream

1 teaspoon garlic-infused olive oil

Salt and freshly ground black pepper

Green salad or vegetables, for serving

---

* You may make your own breadcrumbs by processing gluten-free, soy-free bread into crumbs in a food processor. Breads that include soy lecithin are suitable on the low-FODMAP diet.

Tarragon Chicken Terrine

SERVES 8

A terrine is a savoury loaf made up primarily of meat – in this case chicken, beautifully flavoured with tarragon. Lovely served cold with salad, or as part of an appetizer platter, this dish is sure to please.

1. Preheat the oven to 180°C.
2. Heat the garlic-infused oil, olive oil and butter in a small heavy-bottomed frying pan over medium heat until the butter has melted. Stir in the wine and set aside.
3. Place the chicken thigh meat, ground chicken, bread-crumbs, egg, cream, parsley and tarragon in a large bowl, pour in the wine mixture and mix together well. Season with the salt and pepper.
4. Line a deep 20 x 10 cm loaf tin with overlapping slices of pro-sciutto, leaving a little overhang on both long sides. Spoon the chicken mixture into the tin and smooth the surface. Fold in the over-hanging prosciutto to enclose the filling. Cover the tin with foil and place in a large baking dish. Pour enough boiling water into the dish to come two thirds of the way up the side of the tin.
5. Bake for 1 hour, or until the juices run clear when a tooth-pick is inserted into the centre of the terrine. Set aside to cool to room temperature.
6. Remove the foil and invert the tin onto a wire rack over the baking dish to allow the juices to drain away. After the juices stop running, turn the tin upright and cover again with foil. Top with another loaf tin containing two or three heavy cans, to compress the terrine. Place in the refrigerator for a few hours or overnight.
7. To serve, remove the weights, extra tin and foil, turn out the terrine onto a cutting board, and pat dry with paper towel. Cut into thick slices and serve with your favourite salad.

PER SERVING (not including the green salad): 439 calories; 32 g protein; 27 g total fat; 5 g saturated fat; 15 g carbohydrates; 1 g fibre; 922 mg sodium

2 teaspoons garlic-infused olive oil

2 tablespoons olive oil

30 g salted butter

60 ml dry white wine

400 g boneless, skinless chicken thighs, excess fat removed, finely chopped

340 g minced white meat chicken

Nine 28-g slices gluten-free, soy-free bread, crusts removed, crumbled into coarse crumbs

1 large egg, lightly beaten

125 ml single cream

Small handful of flat-leaf parsley leaves, chopped

Small handful of tarragon leaves, chopped

Salt and freshly ground black pepper

14 long, thin prosciutto slices (about 340 g total)

Boiling water

Green salad, for serving

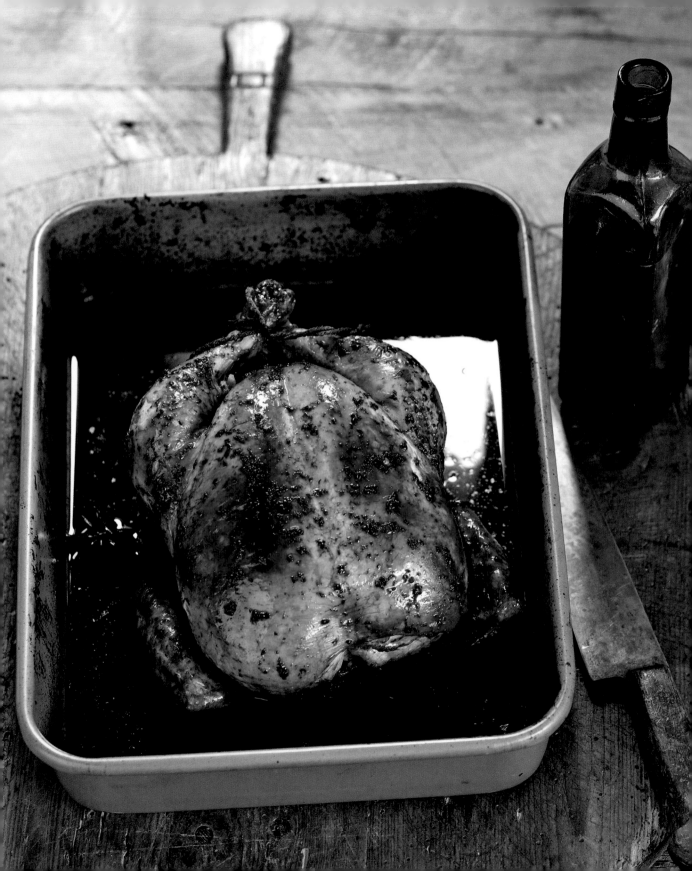

Soy-Infused Roast Chicken

SERVES 4–6

This very fragrant marinade uses a lovely blend of mild aromatic spices. I am sure you will thoroughly enjoy this moist, tender chicken with a subtle infusion of delicious Asian flavours.

1. Combine the soy sauce, sesame oil, brown sugar, ginger, star anise and cinnamon in a bowl and stir until the sugar has dissolved. Place the chicken, breast up, in a roasting pan. Pour the marinade over it and use a pastry brush to ensure the entire chicken is well coated. Cover and refrigerate for 3 to 4 hours, brushing the chicken with the marinade every 1 to 2 hours.

2. Preheat the oven to 180°C.

3. Uncover the chicken, pour the stock into the roasting pan and roast for 30 minutes. Cover loosely with foil and roast for 20 to 30 minutes more, until the juices run clear when you piece the chicken with a toothpick in the thickest part of the thigh. Let rest for a few minutes before carving.

4. Serve with the pan juices and your choice of vegetables.

PER SERVING (⅙ recipe; not including the vegetables): 304 calories; 40 g protein; 12 g total fat; 2 g saturated fat; 6 g carbohydrates; 0 g fibre; 1485 mg sodium

125 ml gluten-free soy sauce

2 tablespoons plus 2 teaspoons sesame oil

2 heaped tablespoons light brown sugar

2 teaspoons grated ginger

3 star anise (or 2 teaspoons ground star anise)

½ teaspoon ground cinnamon

One 1.8-kg whole chicken, excess fat removed

500 ml gluten-free, onion-free chicken stock*

Vegetables, for serving

---

* Most stocks contain onion or garlic. Choose one that is onion-free. If garlic is present, the amount is likely to be minimal and should be suitable for most people on a low-FODMAP diet. If you are extremely sensitive to garlic, omit the stock and use water instead, or make your own stock by boiling chicken bones and/or suitable vegetables (including carrot and celery) in water with your choice of seasonings for about an hour, then straining out the solids.

Swiss Chicken with Mustard Sauce

SERVES 4

This is a great example of a few simple ingredients coming to-gether to create something special. Boneless, skinless chicken breasts work best; make sure you use a sharp kitchen knife to cut them.

1. Cut each chicken breast nearly in half horizontally without cutting all the way through. Open out like a book. Place a piece of cheese and a piece of ham on each, fold the top over the filling, and secure with a toothpick.

2. Set out 3 shallow bowls. Fill one with the cornflour, one with the eggs and one with the breadcrumbs. Beat the eggs lightly. Coat the chicken breasts in the cornflour, shaking off any excess, then dip in the egg and finally toss in the breadcrumbs. Make sure the chicken breasts stay closed, enclosing the filling.

3. Heat the canola oil in a large non-stick pan over medium-low heat. Add the chicken and cook for 4 to 5 minutes on each side, until golden brown and cooked through.

4. Meanwhile, to make the mustard sauce, combine the cream, mayonnaise and mustard in a small saucepan. Stir over medium heat for 3 to 5 minutes, until the sauce has thickened slightly.

5. Divide the chicken among four plates, drizzle with the sauce and serve with your choice of salad or vegetables.

PER SERVING (not including the green salad): 580 calories; 52 g protein; 30 g total fat; 9 g saturated fat; 21 g carbohydrates; 0 g fibre; 622 mg sodium

---

* You may make your own breadcrumbs by processing gluten-free, soy-free bread into crumbs in a food processor. Breads that include soy lecithin are suitable on the low-FODMAP diet.

Four 170-g boneless, skinless chicken breasts

2 slices Swiss cheese, halved

2 slices gluten-free smoked or double-smoked ham, halved

35 g cornflour

2 large eggs

120 g dried gluten-free, soy-free breadcrumbs*

60 ml canola oil

MUSTARD SAUCE

60 ml single cream

75 g gluten-free mayonnaise

2 to 3 teaspoons gluten-free smooth mild mustard

Green salad or vegetables, for serving

Chicken Pockets

I have given you three different fillings to choose from here, but they can all be adapted to suit your taste, so feel free to play around with the ingredients. Each filling recipe makes enough to stuff four chicken breasts, so if you'd like to sample more than one, you'll need to increase the amount of chicken. On a practical note, this is a great way to use up leftover rice.

Four 170-g boneless, skinless chicken breasts

SUN-DRIED TOMATO AND FETA

100 g sun-dried tomatoes, drained (if packed in oil) and finely chopped

150 g cooked white rice

100 g feta, finely diced

1 heaped tablespoon finely grated lemon zest

1 large egg white

2 heaped tablespoons fresh oregano

Salt and freshly ground black pepper

Basting liquid

2 teaspoons garlic-infused olive oil

3 tablespoons olive oil

1 teaspoon fresh oregano

1 teaspoon finely grated lemon zest

MIDDLE EASTERN

170 g mashed sweet potato (from about 1 small sweet potato)

150 g cooked white rice

1 teaspoon ground cumin

1 large egg white

Salt and freshly ground black pepper

Basting liquid

2 teaspoons garlic-infused olive oil

3 tablespoons olive oil

1 teaspoon ground cumin

PESTO

2 heaped tablespoons Basil Pesto (page 64)

150 g cooked white rice

1 large egg white

Salt and freshly ground black pepper

Basting liquid

2 teaspoons garlic-infused olive oil

3 tablespoons olive oil

1 teaspoon Basil Pesto (page 64)

Small basil leaves, for garnish (optional)

Green salad or vegetables, for serving

1. Preheat the oven to 180°C.
2. Using a small sharp knife, insert the blade into the middle of the chicken breast and work to form a pocket (you want to cut to about 1 cm from the internal edge).

(recipe continues)

3. Combine all the ingredients for your choice of filling in a medium bowl and mix well.

4. Spoon the filling into the chicken pockets, pressing it in firmly and making sure it is evenly spread. Seal the ends with a toothpick.

5. Place the chicken breasts on a baking sheet. Whisk together all the ingredients for your choice of basting liquid and brush it over the chicken. Bake for 15 minutes, or until golden brown, then cover with foil and bake for 5 to 10 minutes more, until cooked through (no longer pink inside). Let rest for 5 to 10 minutes.

6. Cut into thick slices, garnish with basil leaves (if desired) and serve with your choice of salad or vegetables.

PER SERVING (not including the green salad):
Sun-Dried Tomato and Feta: 458 calories; 45 g protein; 23 g total fat; 7 g saturated fat; 17 g carbohydrates; 1 g fibre; 597 mg sodium

Middle Eastern: 400 calories; 42 g protein; 15 g total fat; 2 g saturated fat; 22 g carbohydrates; 1 g fibre; 277 mg sodium

Pesto: 393 calories; 42 g protein; 19 g total fat; 3 g saturated fat; 12 g carbohydrates; 0 g fibre; 309 mg sodium

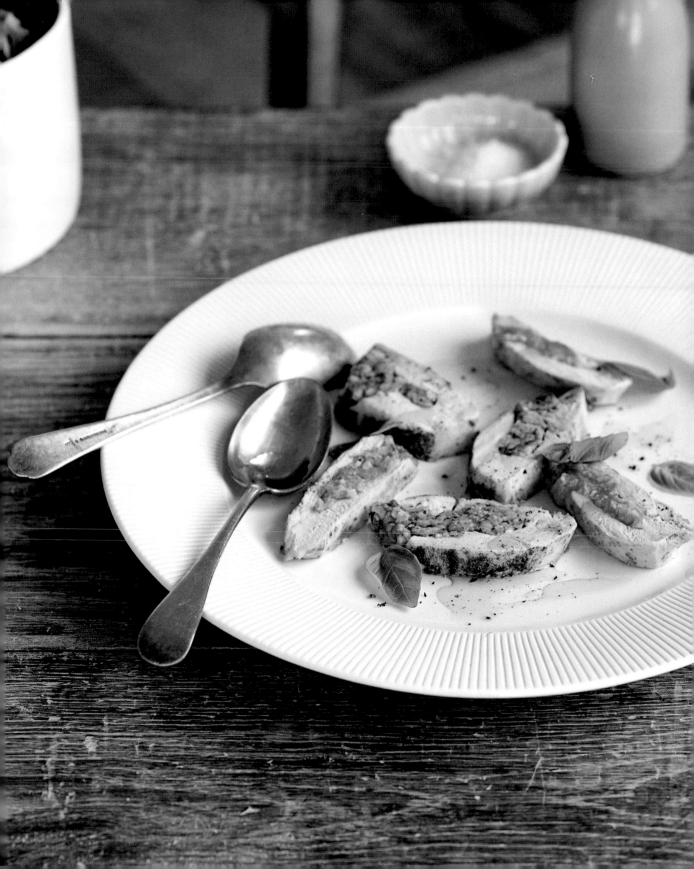

Pork and Vegetable Fricassee with Buttered Quinoa

SERVES 6

Quinoa (pronounced 'keen-wah') is an ancient grain that is packed full of nutrients, and a good source of fibre and plant-based protein. It has a delicious nutty flavour and makes a nice change from traditional potato or rice side dishes. To make this meal vegan, leave out the pork, use vegetable stock and serve double the amount of quinoa (unbuttered) with the vegetable stew.

1. Place the cornflour, salt and pepper in a shallow bowl. Dust the pork in the cornflour, shaking off any excess.

2. Heat the garlic-infused oil and olive oil in a large heavy-bottomed saucepan or stockpot over medium-high heat. Add one third of the pork and cook, stirring, for 2 to 3 minutes, until golden. Transfer to a plate with a slotted spoon and cover to keep warm. Repeat with the remaining pork.

3. Add the tomatoes, tomato passata, carrots, stock and rosemary to the final batch of pork, then return the reserved pork and any juices to the pot. Bring to a boil, then reduce the heat to a simmer. Cover and cook, stirring occasionally, for 1 hour, or until the pork is very tender.

4. Remove the pan from the heat and remove the rosemary stem (the leaves should have cooked off). Stir in the spinach and green beans, then season to taste with salt and pepper. Cook for 5 minutes, or until the beans have softened.

5. Meanwhile, bring a medium saucepan of water to a boil. Add the quinoa and boil for 10 to 12 minutes, until just tender. Drain and rinse under hot water, then drain again. Stir in the butter until melted and season to taste with salt and pepper.

6. Divide the quinoa among shallow bowls and serve with a generous helping of the fricassee.

---

35 g cornflour

Salt and freshly ground black pepper

900 g lean pork, diced

2 teaspoons garlic-infused olive oil

2 teaspoons olive oil

One 400-g tin crushed tomatoes

125 ml tomato passata

2 carrots, sliced

375 ml gluten-free, onion-free beef or vegetable stock*

1 large rosemary sprig

120 g baby spinach leaves

200 g green beans, trimmed and halved

BUTTERED QUINOA

70 g quinoa

15 g salted butter

Salt and freshly ground black pepper

PER SERVING: 409 calories; 36 g protein; 14 g total fat; 5 g saturated fat; 31 g carbohydrates; 6 g fibre; 611 mg sodium

---

* Choose a stock that is onion-free. If garlic is present, the amount is likely to be minimal and should be suitable for most people on a low-FODMAP diet. If you are extremely sensitive to garlic, use water instead, or make your own stock by boiling chicken or beef bones and/or suitable vegetables (including carrot and celery) in water with your choice of seasonings for about an hour, then straining out the solids.

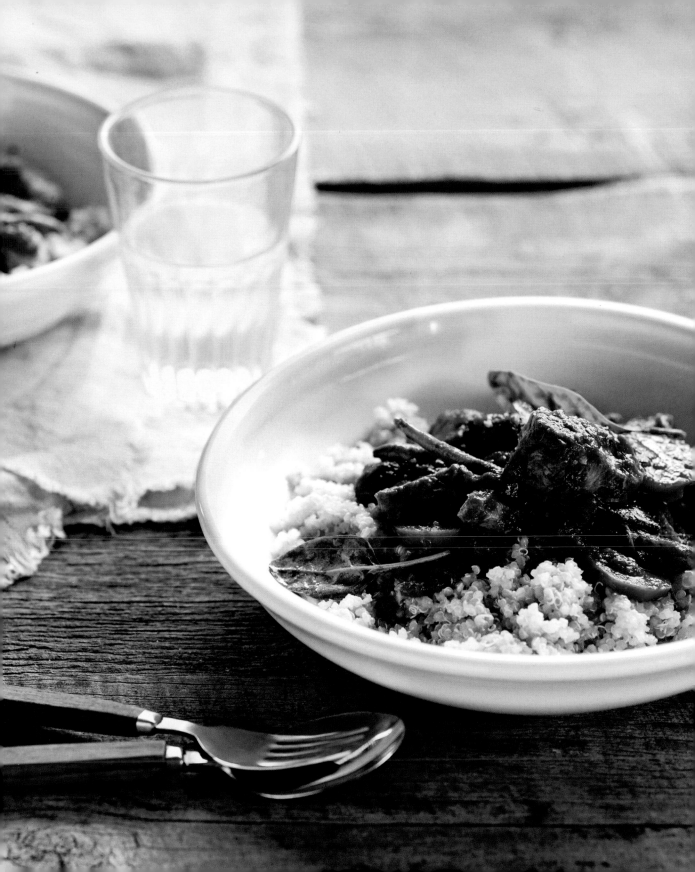

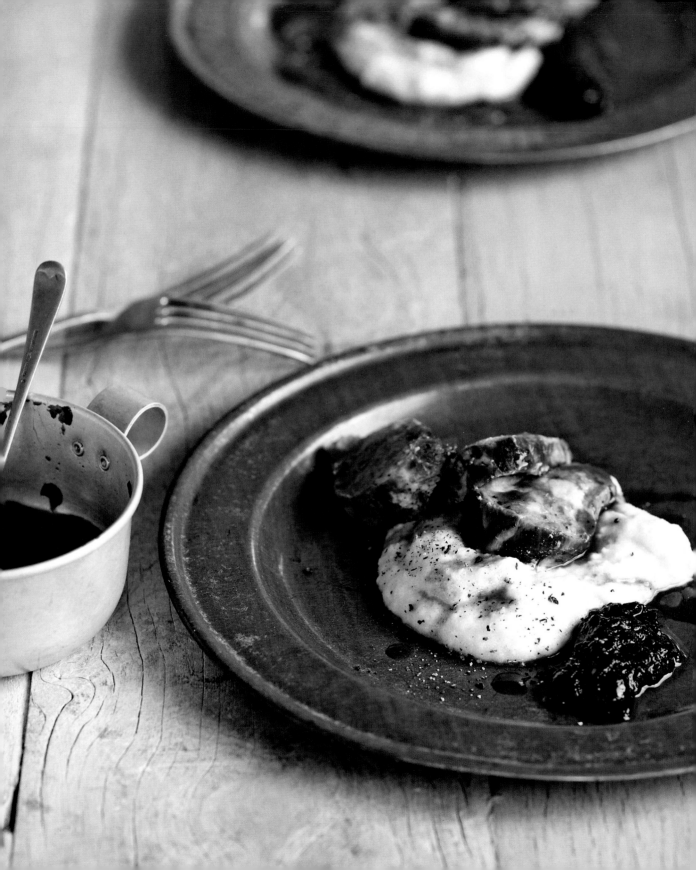

Pork Tenderloin on Creamy Garlic Polenta with Cranberry Sauce

Cranberry sauce isn't just for Thanksgiving! It adds a sweet-tart element to this dish. If you can locate redcurrant jelly, it makes for a nice alternative.

1. Combine the garlic-infused oil, olive oil, lemon juice, salt and pepper in a baking dish. Add the pork and brush the marinade all over. Cover and refrigerate for at least 3 hours.

2. Preheat the oven to 180°C.

3. Remove the pork from the fridge and bake, uncovered, for 30 minutes, or until your desired doneness.

4. Meanwhile, for the polenta, combine the milk and garlic in a medium saucepan over medium heat and bring to just below a boil. Remove the garlic with a slotted spoon and discard. Add the cornmeal and stir until the polenta comes to a boil. Reduce the heat to low and cook, stirring constantly, for 3 to 5 minutes more, until the polenta is the texture of smooth mashed potatoes. Season to taste with salt and pepper.

5. Remove the pork from the baking dish and carefully pour the cooking juices into a small frying pan. Return the pork to the dish and cover with foil to keep warm while you prepare the sauce.

6. Add the cranberry sauce to the cooking juices in the frying pan and cook, stirring, until warmed through and well combined.

7. Cut the pork into thick slices. Spoon the polenta onto warmed plates and top with the pork and a good spoonful of cranberry sauce. Finish with a grinding of pepper and serve with your choice of salad or vegetables.

PER SERVING (not including the green salad): 389 calories; 31 g protein; 15 g total fat; 3 g saturated fat; 33 g carbohydrates; 2 g fibre; 306 mg sodium

1 teaspoon garlic-infused olive oil

1 tablespoon plus 1 teaspoon olive oil

1 tablespoon plus 1 teaspoon fresh lemon juice

Salt and freshly ground black pepper

450 g pork tenderloin

80 g whole berry cranberry sauce

CREAMY GARLIC POLENTA

750 ml semi-skimmed milk, lactose-free milk or suitable plant-based milk

2 garlic cloves, peeled and halved

135 g coarse cornmeal (instant polenta)

Salt and freshly ground black pepper

Green salad or vegetables, for serving

Pork Sausages with Cheesy Potato Rösti

SERVES 4

Many sausages contain onion, sometimes in the form of 'dehydrated vegetables', and gluten in the form of wheat fillers. Happily, gluten-free, onion-free pork sausages are readily available, making this dish a breeze to prepare.

1. Place the potatoes in a medium saucepan and cover with cold water. Bring to a boil over high heat. Reduce the heat to medium-high and boil for 12 to 15 minutes. Test for doneness by inserting a toothpick into the middle of a potato; there should be no resistance. Drain and set aside to cool completely.

2. If making individual rösti, preheat the oven to 120°C.

3. Grate the potatoes into a large bowl and add the butter and salt and pepper to taste. Toss well to combine.

4. Grease a small frying pan with cooking spray and heat over medium heat. Add one quarter of the potatoes and press down firmly. Cook for 15 minutes or until the bottom is golden brown and crisp. Using a spatula, slide the rösti out of the pan onto a cutting board or large plate. Flip it over and return it to the pan. Cook for 10 minutes more, or until cooked through and golden brown. Transfer to a baking sheet and keep warm in the oven while you make the remaining rösti. (Alternatively, make one large rösti in a large frying pan and cut into wedges to serve.)

5. Meanwhile, preheat a ridged grill pan, cast-iron frying pan or grill to medium-high and cook the sausages to your desired doneness.

6. Top each rösti with a slice of Jarlsberg cheese and grill until the cheese has melted. Serve with the sausages, a spoonful of mustard (if desired) and your choice of salad or vegetables.

PER SERVING (not including the mustard and green salad): 662 calories; 22 g protein; 51 g total fat; 23 g saturated fat; 27 g carbohydrates; 4 g fibre; 757 mg sodium

3 or 4 medium russet potatoes (750 g), peeled

45 g salted butter, melted

Salt and freshly ground black pepper

Non-stick cooking spray

Four 70-g gluten-free, onion-free pork sausages

Four 28-g Jarlsberg cheese slices

Gluten-free mustard (optional)

Green salad or vegetables, for serving

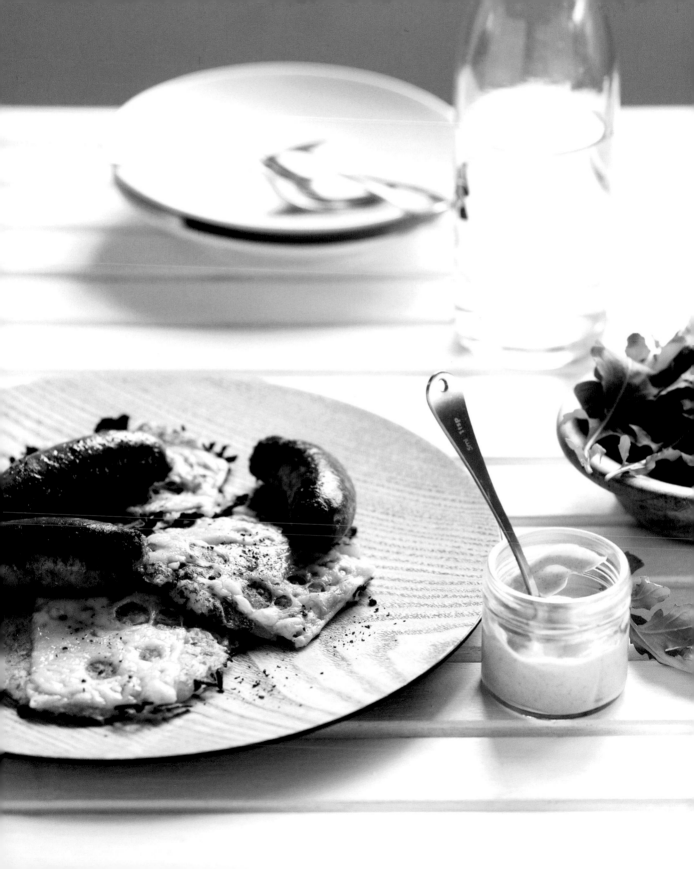

Lime Pork Stir-Fry with Rice Noodles

SERVES 4

Lime leaves add a flavour and freshness to cooking that is unmistakable, so they are worth seeking out in a speciality store or online.

1. Combine the ginger, lime leaves, chilli, lime juice, brown sugar, 1 tablespoon of the soy sauce and 1 tablespoon of the sesame oil in a bowl. Add the pork and toss to coat, then cover and refrigerate for 3 to 4 hours or overnight.

2. Shortly before you're ready to eat, soak the noodles in boiling water for 5 minutes or until tender. Drain and set aside until needed.

3. Heat the remaining 2 tablespoons of sesame oil in a wok, add the pork strips and stir-fry until just cooked.

4. Add the bok choy, red pepper, broccoli and the remaining soy sauce and cook until the vegetables are just tender.

5. Add the noodles and toss to combine. Sprinkle with the coriander and serve.

PER SERVING: 613 calories; 38 g protein; 20 g total fat; 4 g saturated fat; 72 g carbohydrates; 5 g fibre; 1091 mg sodium

1 heaped tablespoon finely grated ginger

6 kaffir lime leaves, shredded, or 1½ heaped tablespoons grated lime zest

1 small red chilli, seeded and thinly sliced

2 tablespoons plus 2 teaspoons fresh lime juice

55 g brown sugar

80 ml gluten-free soy sauce

3 tablespoons sesame oil

600 g lean pork, cut into 3- to 4-mm strips

225 g rice noodles

1 bunch bok choy, leaves separated, cut if large, rinsed and drained

1 red pepper, seeded and cut into thin strips

150 g broccoli florets

5 g roughly chopped coriander

Beef Stir-Fry with Chinese Broccoli and Green Beans

SERVES 4

A stir-fry is a quick and nutritious dinner, perfect for busy weeknights. Marinating the beef will ensure that it is nice and tender.

1. Combine the ginger, garlic-infused oil, olive oil and 2 tablespoons of the sesame oil in a bowl. Add the beef and toss to coat. Cover and refrigerate for 2 to 3 hours.

2. Heat the remaining 2 tablespoons of sesame oil in a wok over medium-high heat. Add the beef and cook for 2 minutes, or until lightly browned. Add the Chinese broccoli, green beans and bean sprouts and stir-fry for 2 to 4 minutes, until the ingredients are tender. Pour in the oyster sauce and cayenne pepper and stir-fry for 1 to 2 minutes, until the sauce is warmed through and the beef and vegetables are coated.

3. Serve over rice or rice noodles.

PER SERVING (not including the rice): 437 calories; 24 g protein; 34 g total fat; 6 g saturated fat; 7 g carbohydrates; 3 g fibre; 92 mg sodium

1 heaped tablespoon grated ginger

2 teaspoons garlic-infused olive oil

2 teaspoons olive oil

60 ml sesame oil

450 g beef sirloin or top round steak, very thinly sliced

1 bunch Chinese broccoli, cut into 3-cm lengths

200 g green beans, trimmed

80 g bean sprouts

1 tablespoon gluten-free, onion-free, garlic-free oyster sauce

¼ teaspoon cayenne pepper

Steamed rice or prepared rice noodles, for serving

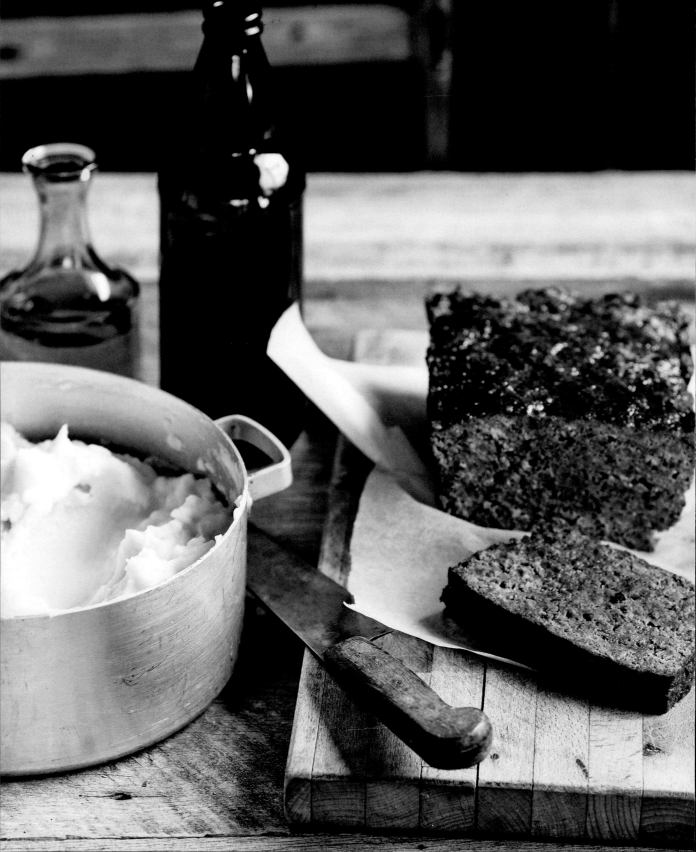

Spanish Meatloaf with Garlic Mashed Potatoes

SERVES 6

Everybody loves meatloaf, and garlic mashed potatoes is its natural partner in crime. Thanks to the garlic-infused oil, there is no garlic in the mashed potatoes, so the dish is safe for everyone to enjoy.

1. Preheat the oven to 180°C. Line a 21.5 x 11.5 cm loaf tin with foil and spray with cooking spray.

2. Combine the beef, tomato purée, breadcrumbs, eggs, garlic-infused oil, olive oil, parsley, ginger, chilli powder, cayenne, paprika, salt and pepper in a large bowl. Mix well with your hands. Press into the loaf tin.

3. Bake for 40 to 45 minutes, until cooked through. (The juices will run clear when you pierce the centre with a small knife.) Let rest for at least 5 minutes before serving.

4. Meanwhile, to make the garlic mashed potatoes, cook the potatoes in a saucepan of boiling water until very tender, about 10 minutes. Drain. Mash with a potato masher. Stir in the garlic-infused oil, butter and milk and season with salt and pepper. Adjust the ingredients for taste or texture if needed.

5. Cut the meatloaf into thick slices and serve with a generous spoonful (or two) of mashed potatoes and your choice of salad or vegetables.

PER SERVING (not including the green salad): 437 calories; 29 g protein; 23 g total fat; 8 g saturated fat; 28 g carbohydrates; 3 g fibre; 370 mg sodium

---

* You may make your own breadcrumbs by processing gluten-free, soy-free bread into crumbs in a food processor. Breads that include soy lecithin are suitable on the low-FODMAP diet.

Non-stick cooking spray

700 g extra-lean minced beef

125 ml tomato purée

90 g dried gluten-free, soy-free breadcrumbs*

2 large eggs, lightly beaten

2 teaspoons garlic-infused olive oil

2 teaspoons olive oil

Small handful of flat-leaf parsley leaves, roughly chopped

¾ teaspoon ground ginger

1 teaspoon chilli powder

1½ teaspoons cayenne pepper

1½ teaspoons sweet paprika

Salt and freshly ground black pepper

GARLIC MASHED POTATOES

4 potatoes, peeled (if desired) and quartered

1 tablespoon garlic-infused olive oil

30 g salted butter

80 ml semi-skimmed milk, lactose-free milk or suitable plant-based milk

Salt and freshly ground black pepper

Green salad or vegetables, for serving

Grilled Steak with Pesto and Potato Wedges

SERVES 4

A step up from steak frites, this is simple, honest food done well. The crunchy herb wedges are divine, and work wonderfully with the basil pesto.

1. Preheat the oven to 200°C. Line a baking sheet with parchment paper.

2. Cut the potatoes in half, then into 1.5-cm wedges. Combine the cornflour, herbs and salt in a resealable plastic bag. Add the potato wedges, seal and toss to coat. Transfer to a colander and shake off any excess coating; the potatoes should only be lightly coated. Place the wedges in a single layer on the baking sheet, brush with the oil, and bake for 10 minutes. Reduce the oven temperature to 180°C and bake for 20 minutes more, turning the wedges halfway through, until crisp and golden brown.

3. Preheat the grill to medium-high, or place a ridged grill pan or cast-iron frying pan over medium-high heat, and cook the steaks to your preferred doneness. Cover and let rest for a few minutes.

4. Serve the steaks and potato wedges with a dollop of pesto.

PER SERVING: 711 calories; 52 g protein; 46 g total fat; 15 g saturated fat; 22 g carbohydrates; 9 g fibre; 498 mg sodium

8 skin-on new potatoes, scrubbed

2 heaped tablespoons cornflour

1 heaped tablespoon finely chopped herbs (such as rosemary and/or oregano)

½ teaspoon salt

2 tablespoons olive oil

900 g beef sirloin or top round steaks, or beef fillet

Basil Pesto (page 64)

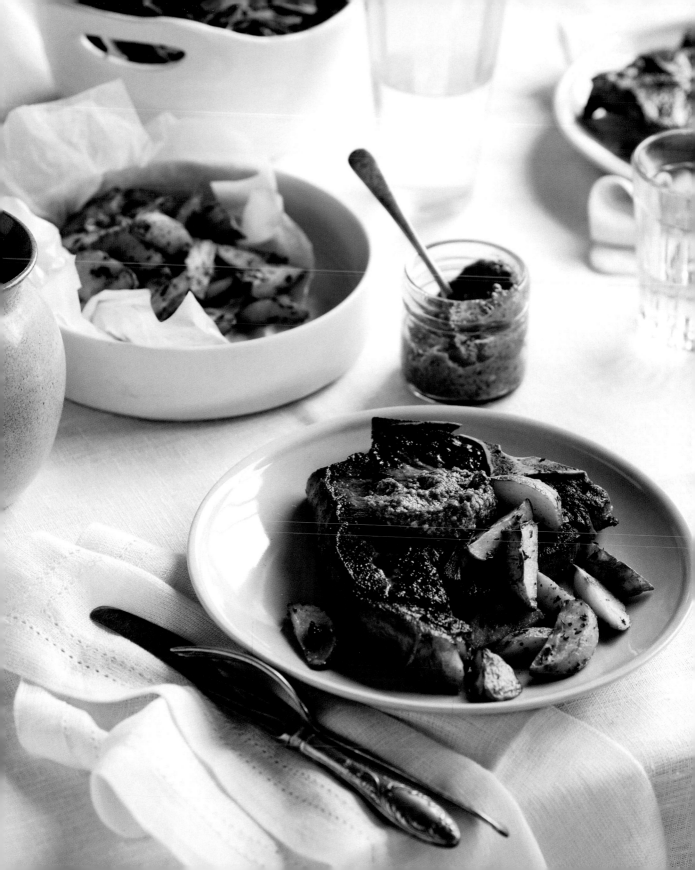

Beef Satay Stir-Fry with Peanut Sauce

SERVES 6–8

If you enjoy Asian food, you're likely familiar with satay sauce. Most versions use onion as a major ingredient, so it was a challenge to recreate the dish without it. After much trial and error, I'm happy with the authentic flavour of this sauce. Unlike the satay you may have eaten on skewers, this version is a stir-fry designed to showcase this low-FODMAP satay sauce.

1. To make the peanut sauce, blend the cornflour with the peanut butter and 2 tablespoons of the stock to make a smooth paste. Stir in the garlic-infused oil, rice bran oil, soy sauce, brown sugar and remaining stock, and season to taste with salt and pepper.

2. Heat the peanut oil in a wok over medium heat. Add one third of the beef and stir-fry until just cooked (it should still be pink on the inside). Remove from the wok and set aside. Cook the remaining beef in two batches and set aside.

3. Add the vegetables to the wok and stir-fry over high heat for 2 to 5 minutes, until just tender, adding a little extra oil if needed. Return the beef and any juices to the wok. Add the sauce and stir-fry until thickened and heated through. Serve with rice.

PER SERVING (⅛ recipe; not including rice): 450 calories; 23 g protein; 32 g total fat; 8 g saturated fat; 19 g carbohydrates; 4 g fibre; 718 mg sodium

* Most stocks contain onion or garlic. Choose one that is onion-free. If garlic is present, the amount is likely to be minimal and should be suitable for most people on a low-FODMAP diet. If you are extremely sensitive to garlic, omit the stock and use water instead, or make your own stock by boiling beef soup bones and/or suitable vegetables (including carrot and celery) in water with your choice of seasonings for about an hour, then straining out the solids.

PEANUT SAUCE

1 heaped tablespoon cornflour

210 g smooth peanut butter

500 ml gluten-free, onion-free beef stock*

2 teaspoons garlic-infused olive oil

2 tablespoons rice bran oil or peanut oil

60 ml gluten-free soy sauce

55 g light brown sugar

Salt and freshly ground black pepper

2 tablespoons peanut oil, plus more if needed

700 g lean beef, sliced 3-mm thick

150 g green beans, trimmed

1 red pepper, seeded and cut into strips

150 g broccoli florets

2 carrots, diced

Steamed rice, for serving

Beef Rolls with Horseradish Cream

SERVES 4

Flank steaks work well for this recipe as they are long and have a fairly consistent width, which is important when rolling them up.

1. Preheat the oven to 180°C. Grease a baking dish with non-stick cooking spray.

2. Place each steak between two sheets of parchment or waxed paper and flatten with a meat tenderiser or rolling pin until the steak is about a third of its original thickness. Cut each steak in half to make 8 thin steaks. Set aside.

3. Mix together the spinach, olives and cream cheese and season with salt and pepper. Place about 1 tablespoon of the cream cheese filling across the centre of each steak portion and roll up to enclose the filling. Secure with a toothpick.

4. Place the rolls in the baking dish and bake for 10 minutes. Cover with foil and bake for 5 minutes more or until cooked through.

5. Meanwhile, to make the horseradish cream, combine all the ingredients in a small saucepan and simmer gently over medium-low heat for 5 to 8 minutes, until thickened slightly. (Don't let it boil.)

6. Serve 2 beef rolls per person with the horseradish cream and your choice of salad or vegetables.

PER SERVING (not including the green salad): 479 calories; 35 g protein; 36 g total fat; 16 g saturated fat; 3 g carbohydrates; 1 g fibre; 391 mg sodium

Non-stick cooking spray

675 g flank, sirloin or top round steak, trimmed of fat and cut into 4 pieces

60 g baby spinach leaves, rinsed, dried and finely chopped

2 heaped tablespoons finely chopped pitted black olives

75 g reduced-fat cream cheese, at room temperature

Salt and freshly ground black pepper

HORSERADISH CREAM

1 heaped tablespoon freshly grated horseradish

Squeeze of fresh lemon juice

60 ml single cream

2 heaped tablespoons finely chopped flat-leaf parsley

Salt and freshly ground black pepper

Green salad or vegetables, for serving

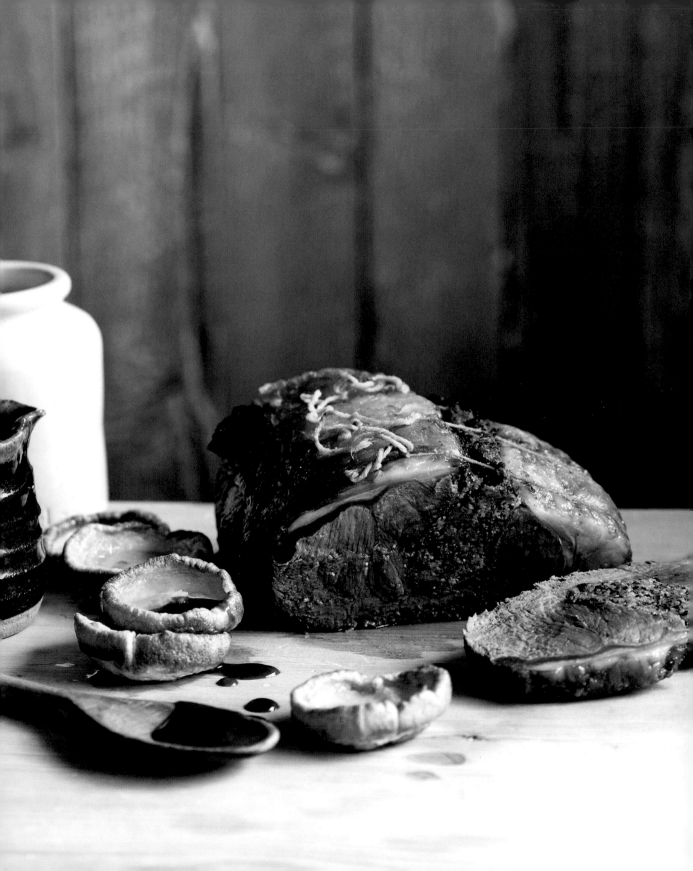

Stuffed Rolled Roast Beef with Yorkshire Puddings and Gravy

SERVES 8

These Yorkshire puddings (also known as popovers in some parts of the world) are traditionally made with white wheat flour, so I'm happy to offer this recipe as a delicious wheat-free alternative. The trick is to have *really* hot oil – so be careful not to spill it and burn yourself.

1. Preheat the oven to 200°C.

2. To make the Yorkshire puddings, sift the rice flour, cornflour and salt three times into a large bowl (or whisk in the bowl until well combined). Make a well in the middle and add the eggs and one third of the milk. Using a wooden spoon, mix the batter from the centre out – first mixing the eggs and milk together, and then gradually working in the flour from the sides. Beat the batter until smooth and shiny. Stir in the remaining milk and let stand for 1 hour.

3. To make the stuffing, combine all the ingredients in a bowl. Set aside.

4. Place the beef on a cutting board and slice horizontally through the thickest part to open out the meat like a book. Press the stuffing along the centre. Carefully roll up the beef to enclose the stuffing and secure with kitchen string at 2-cm intervals.

5. Place the rolled beef in a metal baking dish, seam-side down, brush with the olive oil and sprinkle with the salt. Roast for 40 to 45 minutes for medium-rare, or until your desired doneness. Remove from the oven and increase the oven temperature to 220°C. Transfer the beef to a cutting board and let rest, covered loosely with foil, while you cook the Yorkshire puddings.

6. To cook the Yorkshire puddings, put ½ teaspoon of vegetable oil into each cup of a 12-cup muffin tin. Place on the top shelf of the oven for 5 minutes to heat the oil. Carefully pour the batter into each cup. Reduce the heat to 190°C and bake for 6 to 8 minutes, until they are risen and golden brown.

YORKSHIRE PUDDINGS

65 g superfine white rice flour

50 g cornflour

1 teaspoon salt

2 large eggs

125 ml skimed milk, lactose-free milk or suitable plant-based milk

HERB AND MUSTARD STUFFING

80 g dried gluten-free, soy-free breadcrumbs*

1 large egg

60 ml gluten-free wholegrain mustard

3 to 4 heaped tablespoons roughly chopped flat-leaf parsley

1 heaped tablespoon tomato purée

¼ teaspoon salt

¼ teaspoon freshly ground black pepper

2 teaspoons paprika

1.2 kg beef tenderloin

1 tablespoon olive oil

2 teaspoons salt

2 tablespoons vegetable oil

(recipe and ingredients continue)

7. To make the gravy, combine the pan juices with enough boiling water to equal 250 ml liquid. Return to the baking dish and whisk in the gravy mix. Cook over medium heat, whisking constantly, until thickened and well combined.

8. Remove the string from the beef and slice carefully so you don't disturb the stuffing. Serve with the Yorkshire puddings, gravy and your choice of roasted vegetables.

PER SERVING (not including the roasted vegetables): 578 calories; 31 g protein; 40 g total fat; 15 g saturated fat; 22 g carbohydrates; 0 g fibre; 1205 mg sodium

------

* You may make your own breadcrumbs by processing gluten-free, soy-free bread into crumbs in a food processor. Breads that include soy lecithin are suitable on the low-FODMAP diet. Most gravy mixes contain onion or garlic. Choose one that is onion-free. If garlic is present, the amount is likely to be minimal and should be suitable for most people on a low-FODMAP diet. If you are extremely sensitive to garlic, omit the gravy mix and replace with 1 onion-free beef stock cube (or juice from the roasting pan) and 2 heaped tablespoons cornflour.

GRAVY

About 250 ml boiling water

85 g gluten-free, onion-free gravy mix*

Roasted vegetables, for serving

Rib-Eye Steak with Creamy Prawn Sauce

SERVES 6

Surf and turf at its best! I've suggested rib-eye, but you can choose your favourite cut of steak for this. As always with seafood, try to buy the prawns on the day you want to cook them.

1. Combine the garlic-infused oil, olive oil, lemon juice, salt and pepper in a baking dish. Add the steaks and turn to coat. Cover and refrigerate for at least 3 hours.

2. To make the sauce, blend the cream and cornflour in a small bowl, stirring well to remove any lumps. Heat the garlic-infused oil in a medium frying pan. Add the cream mixture, prawns and parsley and cook until the prawns have turned just pink and the sauce has thickened. Season to taste with salt and pepper.

3. Heat a ridged grill pan, cast-iron frying pan, or grill to medium-high. Cook the steaks to your preferred doneness. Remove from the pan, cover and let rest for a few minutes.

4. Serve the steaks with the prawn sauce and your choice of salad or vegetables.

PER SERVING (not including the green salad): 459 calories; 60 g protein; 25 g total fat; 9 g saturated fat; 2 g carbohydrates; 0 g fibre; 433 mg sodium

2 teaspoons garlic-infused olive oil

2 teaspoons olive oil

1 tablespoon plus 1 teaspoon fresh lemon juice

Salt and freshly ground black pepper

Six 190-g rib-eye steaks (1.125 kg total), trimmed of excess fat

CREAMY PRAWN SAUCE

125 ml single cream

1 teaspoon cornflour

1 teaspoon garlic-infused olive oil

450 g raw jumbo prawns, peeled and deveined, tails intact

2 teaspoons roughly chopped flat-leaf parsley

Salt and freshly ground black pepper

Green salad or vegetables, for serving

Lamb and Vegetable Pilaf

SERVES 4–6

Pilaf makes a nice change from its creamy cousin, risotto. Aromatic spices and crunchy almonds give this dish plenty of flavour and texture. If you'd like to substitute brown basmati rice for the white, you may, but will need to cook the rice longer and use more stock.

1. Heat 1 tablespoon plus 2 teaspoons of the olive oil and the 2 teaspoons garlic-infused oil in a large saucepan or Dutch oven over medium heat. Add the ginger, cinnamon, cloves, cayenne and cumin and cook for 1 to 2 minutes, until fragrant. Add the lamb and toss until browned.

2. Add the rice, sweet potato and aubergine to the pan and cook, stirring, for 2 to 3 minutes, until the rice is well coated in the spiced oil. Pour in the stock and bring to a boil, then reduce the heat to low and simmer, covered, for 10 minutes.

3. Meanwhile, heat the remaining 1 teaspoon of olive oil in a small frying pan over medium heat. Add the almonds and cook, stirring, until golden. Drain on paper towels.

4. Add the courgettes to the rice mixture and cook for 5 minutes more, or until all the liquid has been absorbed and the rice is tender. Remove and discard the whole cloves. Season with salt and pepper, then stir in the almonds, coriander and parsley. Serve hot.

PER SERVING (⅙ recipe): 630 calories; 24 g protein; 34 g total fat; 11 g saturated fat; 54 g carbohydrates; 7 g fibre; 318 mg sodium

2 tablespoons olive oil

2 teaspoons garlic-infused olive oil

2½ teaspoons grated ginger

2 teaspoons ground cinnamon

6 whole cloves

½ teaspoon cayenne pepper

2 teaspoons ground cumin

500 g boneless lamb loin, sliced

300 g white basmati rice

1 small sweet potato, chopped

625 ml gluten-free, onion-free beef or vegetable stock*

65 g slivered almonds

1 large aubergine, trimmed and sliced

2 medium courgettes, halved lengthwise and thickly sliced

Salt and freshly ground black pepper

5 g roughly chopped coriander

3 tablespoons roughly chopped flat-leaf parsley

---

* Most stocks contain onion or garlic. Choose one that is onion-free. If garlic is present, the amount is likely to be minimal and should be suitable for most people on a low-FODMAP diet. If you are extremely sensitive to garlic, omit the stock and use water instead, or make your own stock by boiling beef soup bones and/or suitable vegetables (including carrot and celery) in water with your choice of seasonings for about an hour, then straining out the solids.

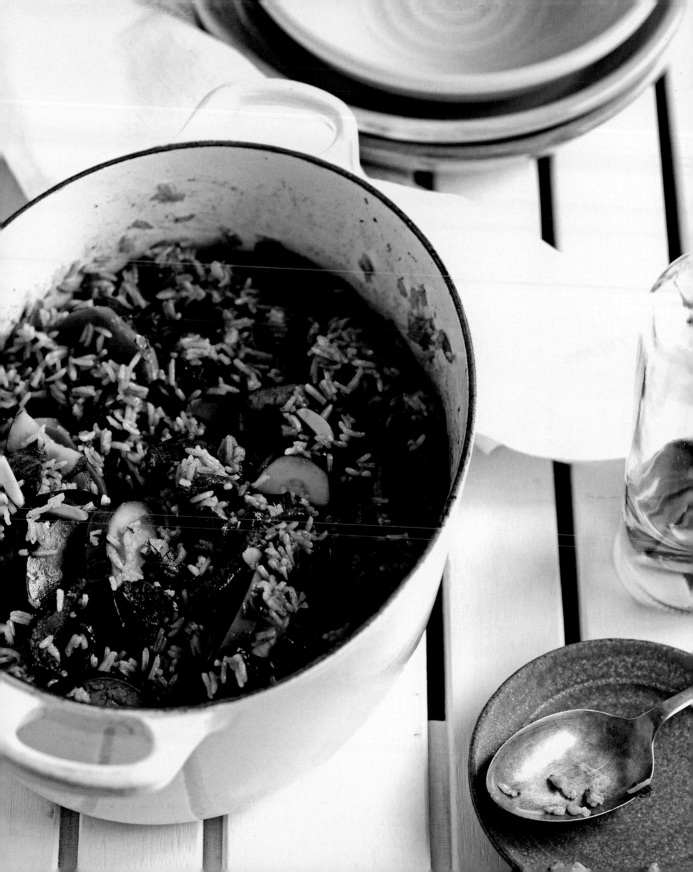

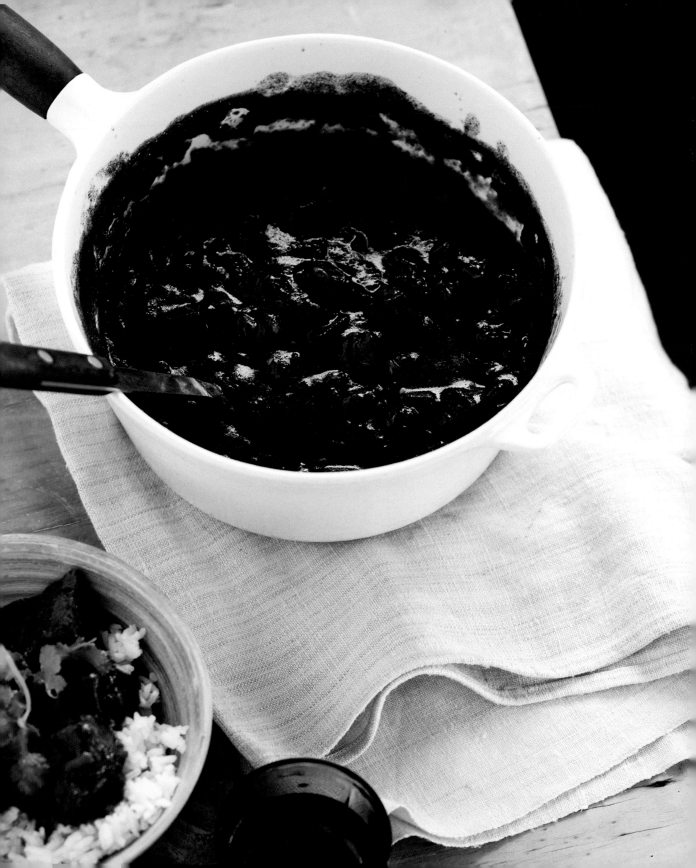

Mild Lamb Curry

SERVES 6–8

Curries at Indian restaurants often include high-FODMAP ingredients such as onions and cream, and may be served with high-FODMAP accompaniments such as pappadum (made with lentil or chickpea flour). This delicious homemade curry, on the other hand, is suitable for anyone following a low-FODMAP diet.

1. Place the cornflour in a shallow bowl. Add the lamb pieces and toss to coat well. Shake off any excess.

2. Heat the garlic-infused oil and rice bran oil in a large heavy-bottomed saucepan or Dutch oven over medium heat. Add the cinnamon, cumin, ginger, turmeric, paprika, cayenne, salt and pepper and cook for 1 to 2 minutes, until fragrant. Add the lamb and cook, stirring occasionally, for 5 to 7 minutes, until nicely browned. Add the stock and brown sugar and bring to a boil, then reduce the heat and simmer gently for 1½ hours, stirring occasionally.

3. Stir in the crushed tomatoes and cook for another hour or until the meat is very tender. Make sure the heat is kept very low so the lamb does not boil dry. (Add a little water if necessary.)

4. Season to taste with salt and pepper and serve with steamed rice, garnished with coriander.

PER SERVING (⅛ recipe; not including rice or coriander): 538 calories; 27 g protein; 39 g total fat; 15 g saturated fat; 16 g carbohydrates; 2 g fibre; 647 mg sodium

---

* Most stocks contain onion or garlic. Choose one that is onion-free. If garlic is present, the amount is likely to be minimal and should be suitable for most people on a low-FODMAP diet. If you are extremely sensitive to garlic, omit the stock and use water instead, or make your own stock by boiling beef soup bones and/or suitable vegetables (including carrot and celery) in water with your choice of seasonings for about an hour, then straining out the solids.

75 g cornflour

1.2 kg lean lamb steaks, cut into 2-cm pieces

2 teaspoons garlic-infused olive oil

2 tablespoons rice bran oil or sunflower oil

2 teaspoons ground cinnamon

2 heaped tablespoons ground cumin

2 teaspoons ground ginger

1 heaped tablespoon ground turmeric

2 teaspoons paprika

1 teaspoon cayenne pepper

1 teaspoon salt

1 teaspoon freshly ground black pepper

1 litre gluten-free, onion-free beef stock*

2 heaped tablespoons light brown sugar

One 425-g can crushed tomatoes

Steamed rice and coriander leaves, for serving

Roasted Lamb Racks on Buttered Mashed Swede

SERVES 4–8

Mashed swede makes a nice change from mashed potato, and tastes so good with a dab of butter stirred in. Serve with a variety of other vegetables, if you wish.

1. Preheat the oven to 180°C.
2. Combine the butter, cumin, salt and pepper in a small bowl. Rub over the lamb racks. Place the lamb in a baking dish and roast for 30 minutes or until the lamb is cooked but still pink in the middle. Remove from the oven and let rest for a few minutes.
3. Meanwhile, to make the mashed swede, cook the swede in boiling water for 8 to 10 minutes, until tender. Drain, then mash with a potato masher. Stir in the butter while still hot, and season well with salt and pepper.
4. Cut each rack of lamb in half or in quarters and serve on a bed of mashed swede.

PER SERVING (⅛ recipe): 448 calories; 26 g protein; 31 g total fat; 14 g saturated fat; 16 g carbohydrates; 5 g fibre; 650 mg sodium

30 g salted butter, at room temperature

1 teaspoon ground cumin

Salt and freshly ground black pepper

2 lamb racks (8 chops each, about 1.3 g total), trimmed of fat

BUTTERED MASHED SWEDE

2 large swede (800 g total), peeled and cut into 5-cm chunks

15 g salted butter, at room temperature

Salt and freshly ground black pepper

DESSERTS

Almond Biscuits

MAKES ABOUT 40

These biscuits, a gluten-free variation on a recipe from my childhood, have a wonderfully light and slightly chewy texture.

1. Preheat the oven to 140°C. Line two baking sheets with parchment paper.

2. Combine the almond flour, cornflour and baking powder in a small bowl. Beat the egg white in a clean medium bowl with a handheld electric mixer until soft peaks form. Gradually beat in the sugar. Continue beating for 5 minutes more or until stiff peaks form. Add the almond flour mixture, lemon zest, almond extract and melted butter and gently mix together with a large metal spoon.

3. Roll 2 teaspoons of the dough into a ball. Repeat with the remaining dough to make about 40 balls, placing them on the baking sheets and leaving a little room for spreading. Flatten slightly. Bake for 25 minutes, until they have started turning a light golden brown.

4. Cool on the sheets for 5 minutes, then transfer to a wire rack to cool completely.

PER SERVING: 25 calories; 1 g protein; 1 g total fat; 0 g saturated fat; 3 g carbohydrates; 0 g fibre; 7 mg sodium

90 g almond flour

1 tablespoon plus 1 teaspoon cornflour

½ teaspoon gluten-free baking powder

1 large egg white

110 g caster sugar

1 teaspoon finely grated lemon zest

3 drops almond extract

15 g unsalted butter, melted

Peanut Butter and Sesame Biscuits

MAKES 20–25

Although the name of these biscuits might lead you to believe they are savoury, they are in fact mildly sweet. They make a delicious change from the usual sweet biscuit flavours.

1. Preheat the oven to 170°C. Line two baking sheets with parchment paper.

2. Place the butter, peanut butter, brown sugar and caster sugar in a medium bowl and beat with a handheld electric mixer until creamy. Add the eggs, vanilla and sesame seeds and beat well.

3. Sift the rice flour, cornflour, soy flour, baking soda and xanthan gum three times into a large bowl (or whisk in the bowl until well combined). Add to the peanut butter mixture and mix with a large metal spoon until well combined.

4. Shape the dough into walnut-size balls and place on the sheets, leaving a little room for spreading. Gently flatten to about 5 mm thick.

5. Bake for 10 to 12 minutes, until golden.

6. Cool on the sheets for 5 minutes, then transfer to a wire rack to cool completely.

PER SERVING (¹⁄₂₅ **recipe**): 130 calories; 5 g protein; 7 g total fat; 2 g saturated fat; 13 g carbohydrates; 1 g fibre; 84 mg sodium

30 g unsalted butter, at room temperature

280 g smooth peanut butter

55 g light brown sugar

2 heaped tablespoons caster sugar

2 large eggs, lightly beaten

1 teaspoon vanilla extract

35 g sesame seeds

85 g superfine white rice flour

110 g cornflour

45 g soy flour

½ teaspoon baking soda

1 teaspoon xanthan gum or guar gum

Hazelnut or Almond Crescents

MAKES ABOUT 40

If you're looking for a little sweet something to enjoy with a cup of tea or coffee, these half-moon-shaped biscuits are just the thing. They also make a lovely gift at Christmas time – or any time, really!

1. Sift the rice flour and cornflour into a medium bowl (or whisk in the bowl until well combined). Stir in the caster sugar and hazelnut flour. Rub in the butter with your fingertips until the mixture resembles breadcrumbs. Mix in the egg yolk and vanilla with a large metal spoon.

2. Lightly sprinkle your work surface with rice flour. Gently press the dough into a ball, turn out onto the floured surface and knead lightly until smooth. Divide the dough into two even portions, wrap each in cling film, and refrigerate for 15 minutes.

3. While the dough is chilling, preheat the oven to 160°C. Line two baking sheets with parchment paper.

4. Unwrap the dough and roll each portion into a log with a diameter of about 2 cm. Cut 2-to 3-cm slices and shape them into rounded crescents with your hands. Place on the baking sheets, leaving room for spreading.

5. Bake for 15 to 20 minutes, until lightly golden. Let cool on the sheets for 5 minutes.

6. Sift the icing sugar into a shallow bowl (or whisk well in the bowl). Roll the warm biscuits in the sugar until well coated, then transfer to a wire rack to cool completely. Dust with extra icing sugar just before serving.

45 g superfine white rice flour, plus more for the work surface

35 g cornflour

55 g caster sugar

125 g hazelnut or almond flour

105 g unsalted butter, cut into cubes, at room temperature

1 large egg yolk, at room temperature, lightly beaten

1 teaspoon vanilla extract

80 g icing sugar, plus more for dusting

PER SERVING:

Almond: 57 calories; 1 g protein; 4 g total fat; 1 g saturated fat; 5 g carbohydrates; 0 g fibre; 2 mg sodium

Hazelnut: 60 calories; 1 g protein; 4 g total fat; 1 g saturated fat; 5 g carbohydrates; 0 g fibre; 0 mg sodium

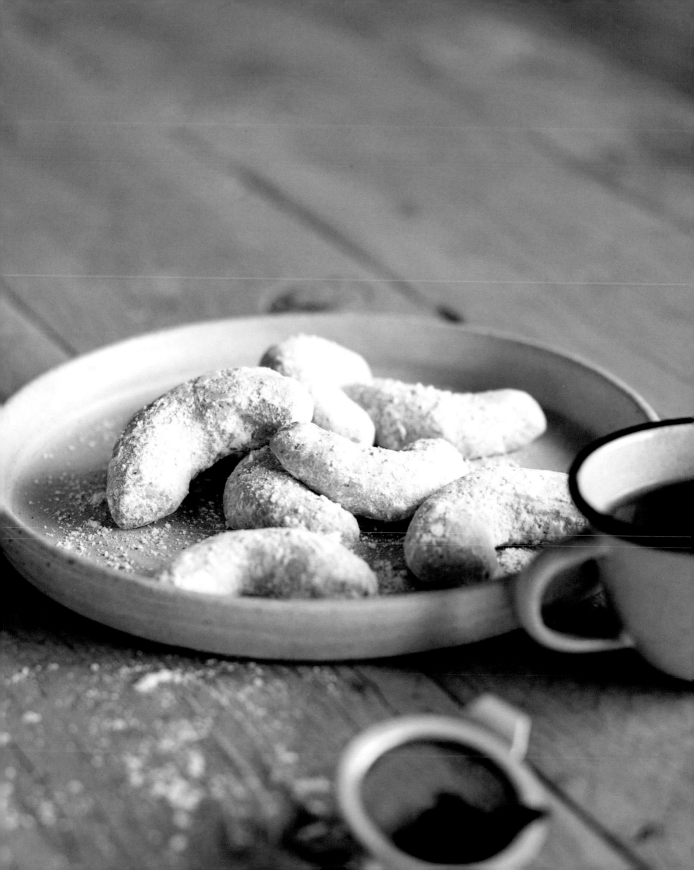

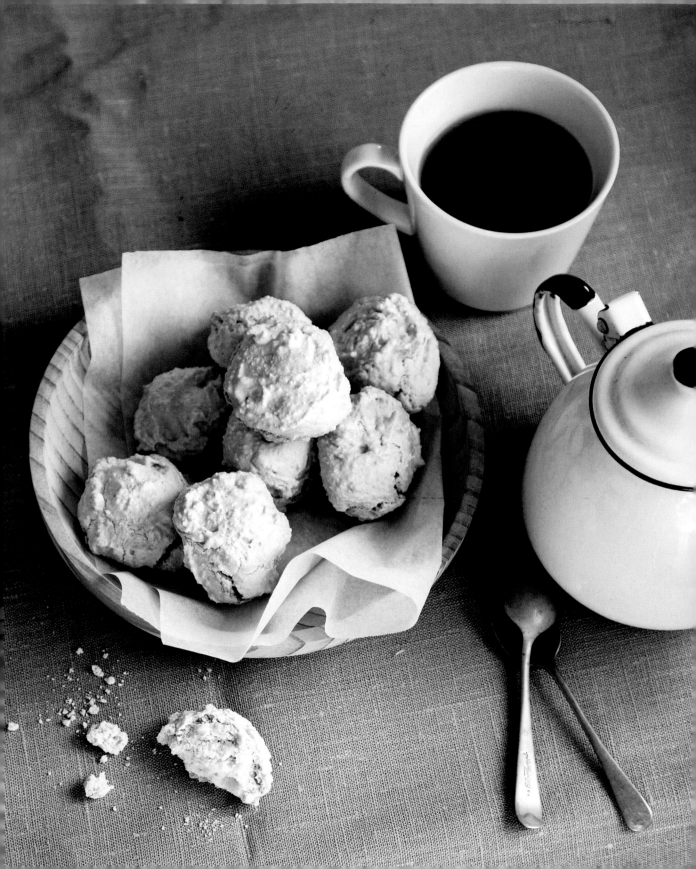

Amaretti

MAKES 20–25

These crisp biscuits have a delicate marzipan flavour. They taste great on their own, but they can also be used in dessert recipes. Try them in the tiramisu on page 191.

1. Preheat the oven to 170°C. Line two baking sheets with parchment paper.

2. Place the almond flour, icing sugar and cornflour in a medium bowl and mix together well.

3. Beat the egg whites in a clean medium bowl with a hand-held electric mixer until soft peaks form. Add the caster sugar, 1 tablespoon at a time, and beat until shiny and stiff peaks form. Add the almond extract and beat to combine well. Gently fold in the almond flour mixture with a large metal spoon until just blended.

4. Place rounded teaspoons of the batter on the baking sheets, leaving room for spreading. Smooth the top of each cookie with the back of a metal spoon. Bake for 18 to 25 minutes, until lightly golden. Turn off the oven, leave the door ajar and let the biscuits cool and dry out in the oven.

PER SERVING (1/25 recipe): 53 calories; 1 g protein; 2 g total fat; 0 g saturated fat; 8 g carbohydrates; 0 g fibre; 6 mg sodium

120 g almond flour
(preferably finely ground)

120 g icing sugar

1 tablespoon plus 1 teaspoon cornflour

2 large egg whites

75 g caster sugar

1 teaspoon almond extract

Banana Friands
(Mini Almond Cakes)

MAKES 12

Friands are small French cakes made with almond flour. They are often made without other flour, but both of my recipes use a small amount of gluten-free flour to give the cakes a nice light texture.

1. Preheat the oven to 180°C. Lightly grease a 12-cup muffin tin, friand pan or petite loaf pan with cooking spray.

2. Melt the butter in a small saucepan over low heat, then cook for 3 to 4 minutes more, until flecks of brown appear. Set aside.

3. Sift the icing sugar, cornflour and rice flour three times into a large bowl (or whisk in the bowl until well combined). Stir in the almond flour, then add the egg whites, lemon juice, vanilla and melted butter and mix with a large metal spoon until combined. Stir in the chopped banana.

4. Spoon the batter into the tin until each cup is two-thirds full. Bake for 12 to 15 minutes, until lightly golden and firm to the touch (a toothpick inserted into the centre should come out clean).

5. Cool in the pan for 5 minutes, then turn out onto a wire rack to cool completely. Dust with icing sugar before serving.

PER SERVING: 229 calories; 4 g protein; 15 g total fat; 6 g saturated fat; 22 g carbohydrates; 2 g fibre; 29 mg sodium

Non-stick cooking spray

135 g unsalted butter, cut into cubes

200 g icing sugar, plus more for dusting

35 g cornflour

35 g superfine white rice flour

150 g almond flour

5 large egg whites, lightly beaten

1 tablespoon plus 1 teaspoon fresh lemon juice

1 teaspoon vanilla extract

1 small ripe banana, peeled and roughly chopped

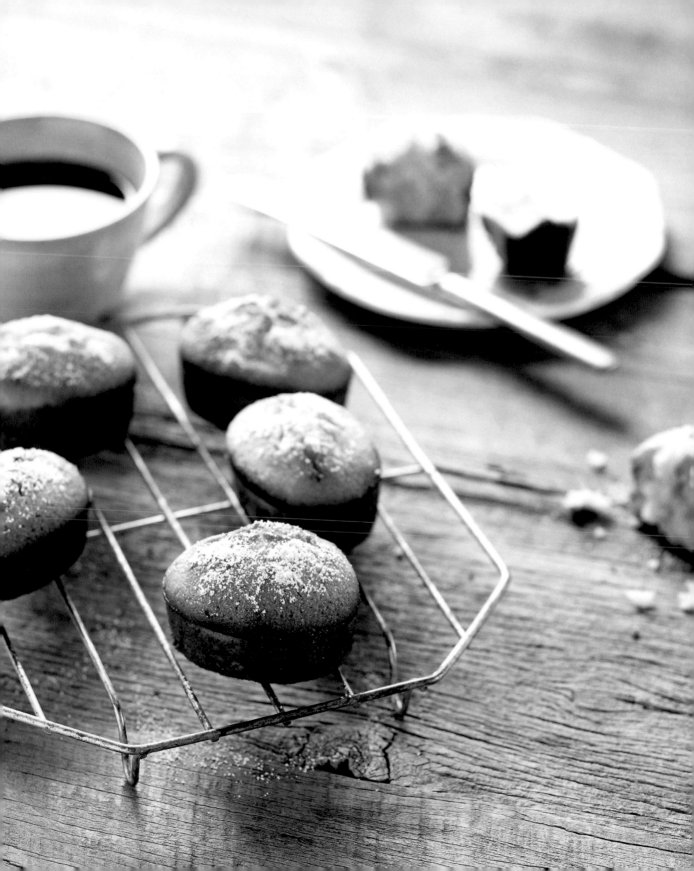

Berry Friands
(Mini Almond Cakes)

MAKES 12

You can use fresh or frozen berries when making these friands; if you are using frozen, add them straight from the freezer so the juices don't run as they thaw. Tinned fruit doesn't tend to work as well because the fruit often splits and stains the batter.

1. Preheat the oven to 180°C. Lightly grease a 12-cup muffin tin, friand pan or petite loaf pan with cooking spray.

2. Melt the butter in a small saucepan over low heat, then cook for 3 to 4 minutes more, until flecks of brown appear. Set aside.

3. Sift the icing sugar, cornflour and rice flour three times into a large bowl (or whisk in the bowl until well combined). Stir in the almond flour, then add the egg whites, lemon juice, vanilla and melted butter and mix with a large metal spoon until combined.

4. Spoon the batter into the tin until each cup is two-thirds full. Gently press about 4 berries into the centre of each friand (without pressing all the way into the batter). Bake for 12 to 15 minutes, until lightly golden and firm to the touch (a toothpick inserted into the centre should come out clean).

5. Cool in the pan for 5 minutes, then turn out onto a wire rack to cool completely. Dust with icing sugar before serving.

PER SERVING (with blueberries): 237 calories; 4 g protein; 15 g total fat; 6 g saturated fat; 24 g carbohydrates; 2 g fibre; 29 mg sodium

Non-stick cooking spray

135 g unsalted butter, cut into cubes

240 g icing sugar, plus more for dusting

35 g cornflour

35 g superfine white rice flour

150 g almond flour

5 large egg whites, lightly beaten

1 tablespoon plus 1 teaspoon fresh lemon juice

2 teaspoons vanilla extract

150 g blueberries or raspberries

Banana Fritters with Fresh Pineapple

SERVES 4

Banana fritters take me straight back to my childhood. For this more grown-up recipe, I've lightened the texture a bit by using sweetened breadcrumbs instead of batter, and served them with fresh, low-FODMAP tropical fruit. Completely delicious, if I do say so myself!

1. Preheat the oven to 150°C.
2. Combine the breadcrumbs, brown sugar and cinnamon on a large plate. Lightly beat the eggs with the icing sugar in a shallow bowl.
3. Dip the banana halves into the egg mixture, then toss in the breadcrumbs until well coated.
4. Melt 1 tablespoon of the butter in a large non-stick frying pan over medium-low heat. Add half of the banana pieces and cook for 3 to 4 minutes on each side, until golden brown. Transfer to a baking sheet and keep warm in the oven. Melt the remaining 1 tablespoon butter and cook the remaining banana halves the same way.
5. Place two banana halves each on four plates. Top with ice cream, pineapple and passion fruit pulp (if desired). Serve immediately.

PER SERVING (with optional passion fruit; not including ice cream): 357 calories; 6 g protein; 9 g total fat; 5 g saturated fat; 66 g carbohydrates; 6 g fibre; 74 mg sodium

---

* You may make your own breadcrumbs by processing gluten-free, soy-free bread into crumbs in a food processor. Breads that include soy lecithin are suitable on the low-FODMAP diet.

120 g dried gluten-free, soy-free breadcrumbs*

75 g light brown sugar

1 tablespoon ground cinnamon

2 large eggs

½ teaspoon icing sugar

4 small bananas, peeled and halved lengthwise

30 g unsalted butter

Gluten-free, lactose-free vanilla ice cream, for serving

½ small pineapple, peeled, cored and finely chopped

Pulp of 2 passion fruits (optional)

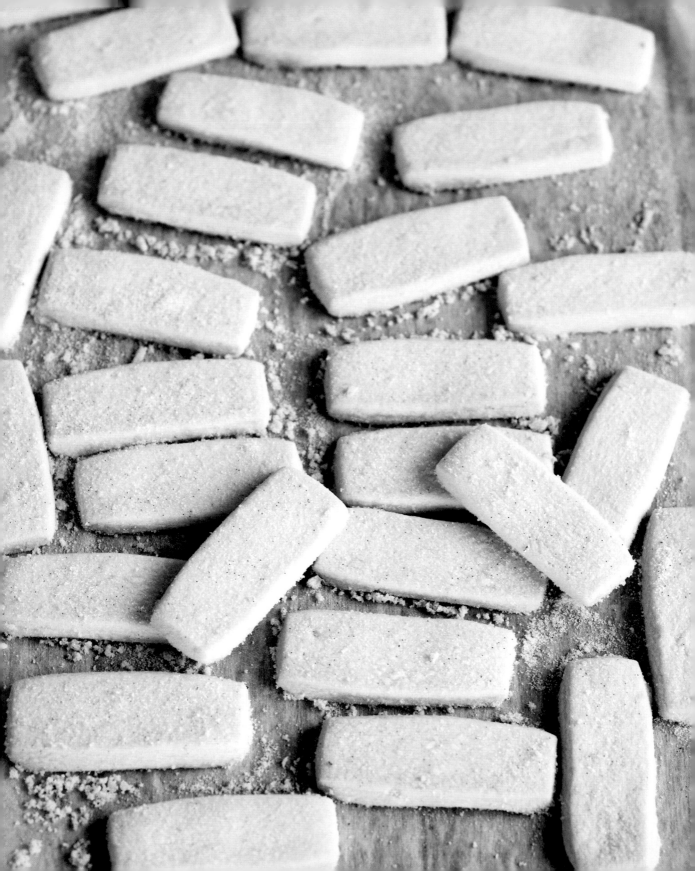

Shortbread Fingers

MAKES ABOUT 36

As you might expect, vanilla sugar is sugar flavoured with vanilla. It is available in the baking section of the supermarket, but if you can't find it, make a batch of your own by burying the scraped seeds and empty pod of a vanilla bean in 450 g caster sugar and letting sit, tightly sealed, for a week or two. If you're in a time pinch, you can also replace it with regular sugar (ideally caster) and add 1 teaspoon vanilla extract to the shortbread dough.

160 g icing sugar

1 tablespoon plus 2 teaspoons vanilla sugar, plus more for sprinkling

300 g cornflour, plus more for kneading

90 g soy flour

65 g superfine white rice flour

2 teaspoons xanthan gum or guar gum

255 g unsalted butter, cut into cubes, at room temperature

1. Preheat the oven to 130°C. Line two baking sheets with parchment paper.

2. Place the icing sugar, vanilla sugar, cornflour, soy flour, rice flour and xanthan gum in a food processor or blender and process until well combined. Add the butter and process for 3 to 5 minutes more to bring together into a dough.

3. Lightly sprinkle your work surface with cornflour. Turn out the dough onto the surface and knead gently until it holds together.

4. Roll out the dough between two sheets of parchment paper to a thickness of 1.25 cm. Cut into 5 x 2 cm rectangles and place on the baking sheets, leaving a little room for spreading. Sprinkle with a little extra vanilla sugar.

5. Bake for 20 to 25 minutes, until golden. Reduce the temperature to 100°C and bake for 10 minutes more, until the shortbread is turning a light golden colour.

6. Cool on the sheets for 10 to 12 minutes, then transfer to a wire rack to cool completely.

PER SERVING: 106 calories; 2 g protein; 5 g total fat; 3 g saturated fat; 13 g carbohydrates; 0 g fibre; 6 mg sodium

Caramel Nut Bars

SERVES 18–20

Xanthan gum binds together the crust of these nutty, gooey bars. It can be found in health food shops or the health food or baking sections of well-stocked supermarkets.

1. Preheat the oven to 180°C. Grease a 28 x 18 cm baking tin with cooking spray and line with parchment paper, leaving an overhang on the two long sides to help lift out the bars later.

2. Sift the rice flour, potato flour, cornflour, caster sugar, baking soda, baking powder and xanthan gum together three times into a bowl (or whisk in the bowl until well combined). Rub in the butter with your fingertips. Add the egg and vanilla and mix with a large metal spoon until well combined. As the mixture becomes more solid, use your hands to bring it together to form a ball.

3. Roll out the dough between two sheets of parchment paper to a thickness of 5 mm. Gently fit into the bottom of the tin and prick all over with a fork. Refrigerate for 10 minutes.

4. Bake for 10 to 12 minutes, until the crust is firm and lightly golden. Set aside to cool, but leave the oven on.

5. To make the topping, combine the brown sugar and butter in a large saucepan over medium heat and stir until the butter has melted and the mixture comes to a boil. Remove from the heat and stir in the cream and cornflour, mixing until smooth. Add the pecans, Brazil nuts and macadamia nuts. Return the pan to medium heat and stir until the mixture comes to a boil. Reduce the heat to low and cook gently for 2 to 3 minutes more, until the mixture is thick and sticky.

6. Spread the nut topping evenly over the crust and bake for 15 minutes, or until the topping is bubbling. Let cool completely in the tin, then transfer to a board, remove the parchment paper, and cut into small (or large!) pieces to serve.

PER SERVING ($\frac{1}{20}$ **recipe**): 278 calories; 3 g protein; 20 g total fat; 8 g saturated fat; 25 g carbohydrates; 1 g fibre; 39 mg sodium

Non-stick cooking spray

65 g superfine white rice flour

45 g potato flour

50 g cornflour

55 g caster sugar

¼ teaspoon baking soda

¼ teaspoon gluten-free baking powder

1 teaspoon xanthan gum or guar gum

60 g unsalted butter, cut into cubes, at room temperature

1 large egg, beaten

1 teaspoon vanilla extract

NUT TOPPING

220 g light brown sugar

150 g unsalted butter, cut into cubes, at room temperature

80 ml single cream

3 tablespoons plus 1 teaspoon cornflour

65 g roasted unsalted pecans, roughly chopped

110 g roasted unsalted Brazil nuts (skin on), roughly chopped

70 g roasted unsalted macadamia nuts, halved

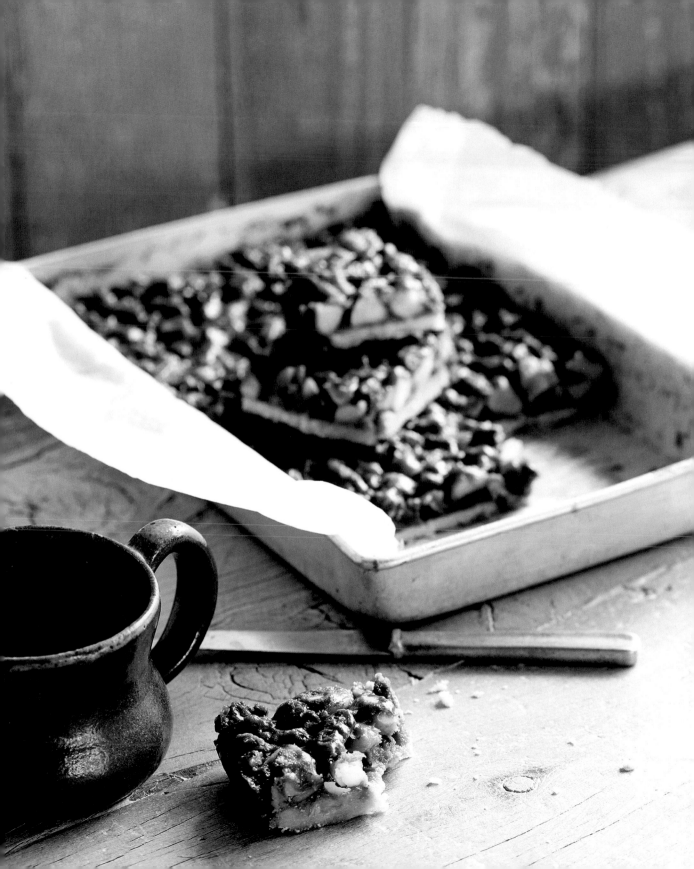

Chocolate-Mint Bars

SERVES 18–20

The chocolate-mint combination is an oldie but a goodie. These delicious bars are always a hit at parties and other social gatherings. Any leftovers will keep well in the fridge for up to a week.

1. Preheat the oven to 170°C. Grease a 29 × 19 cm baking tin with non-stick cooking spray and line with parchment paper.

2. Combine the butter and sugar in a medium bowl and beat with a handheld electric mixer until thick and pale.

3. Sift the rice flour, soy flour, cornflour, xanthan gum and cocoa three times into a separate bowl (or whisk in a bowl until well combined). Add to the creamed butter and sugar and stir with a large metal spoon until well combined. Gently gather into a ball and knead lightly in the bowl. Press the dough into the prepared tin.

4. Bake for 10 to 15 minutes, until lightly browned. Set aside to cool completely.

5. To make the peppermint filling, combine the icing sugar, cream cheese and peppermint extract in a bowl and beat with a handheld electric mixer until well combined. Add the shortening and beat for 1 to 2 minutes, until smooth. Spread the filling evenly over the biscuit crust and refrigerate until set.

6. To make the chocolate topping, combine the dark chocolate, cream and shortening in a small saucepan and stir over low heat until melted and well combined.

7. Remove the pan from the refrigerator and spread the chocolate topping over the peppermint filling. Refrigerate until set, then cut into squares to serve.

PER SERVING (1/20 **recipe**): 247 calories; 2 g protein; 19 g total fat; 9 g saturated fat; 19 g carbohydrates; 1 g fibre; 42 mg sodium

Non-stick cooking spray

120 g unsalted butter, cut into cubes, at room temperature

75 g caster sugar

65 g superfine white rice flour

20 g soy flour

75 g cornflour

1 teaspoon xanthan gum or guar gum

2 heaped tablespoons unsweetened cocoa powder

PEPPERMINT FILLING

160 g icing sugar

One 225 g packet reduced-fat cream cheese, at room temperature

3 to 4 teaspoons peppermint extract

120 g vegetable shortening, melted

CHOCOLATE TOPPING

115 g good-quality dark chocolate, broken into pieces

1 tablespoon plus 1 teaspoon single cream

30 g vegetable shortening

Dark Chocolate–Macadamia Nut Brownies

SERVES 18–20

For best results with these brownies, I urge you to use superfine rice flour (available from Asian grocers, the Asian section of larger supermarkets or online). Regular rice flour is too grainy and won't work nearly as well.

1. Preheat the oven to 160°C. Grease a 29 × 19 cm baking tin with cooking spray and line with parchment paper.

2. Combine the butter and chocolate in a medium saucepan over low heat and stir until melted and smooth. Add the brown sugar and stir until dissolved. Transfer to a large bowl and let cool to room temperature.

3. Sift the rice flour, cornflour and xanthan gum three times into a separate bowl (or whisk in a bowl until well combined).

4. Stir the eggs into the chocolate mixture, one at a time. Add the sifted flour mixture, vanilla, chocolate chips, cream and macadamia nuts (if using). Mix well, spoon into the baking tin, and smooth the surface.

5. Bake for 20 minutes, then cover with foil and bake for 20 to 25 minutes more, until just firm to the touch.

6. Remove from the oven and let cool in the tin to room temperature. Transfer to the refrigerator for 2 to 3 hours or overnight, until firm.

7. Turn out onto a cutting board, peel off the parchment paper and cut into squares to serve.

PER SERVING [$\frac{1}{20}$ recipe): 278 calories; 3 g protein; 18 g total fat; 9 g saturated fat; 31 g carbohydrates; 2 g fibre; 23 mg sodium

Non-stick cooking spray

150 g unsalted butter, cut into cubes

300 g good-quality dark chocolate, broken into pieces

275 g light brown sugar

85 g superfine white rice flour

35 g cornflour

1 teaspoon xanthan gum or guar gum

3 large eggs

2 teaspoons vanilla extract

95 g dark chocolate chips

125 ml single cream

100 g roughly chopped macadamia nuts (optional)

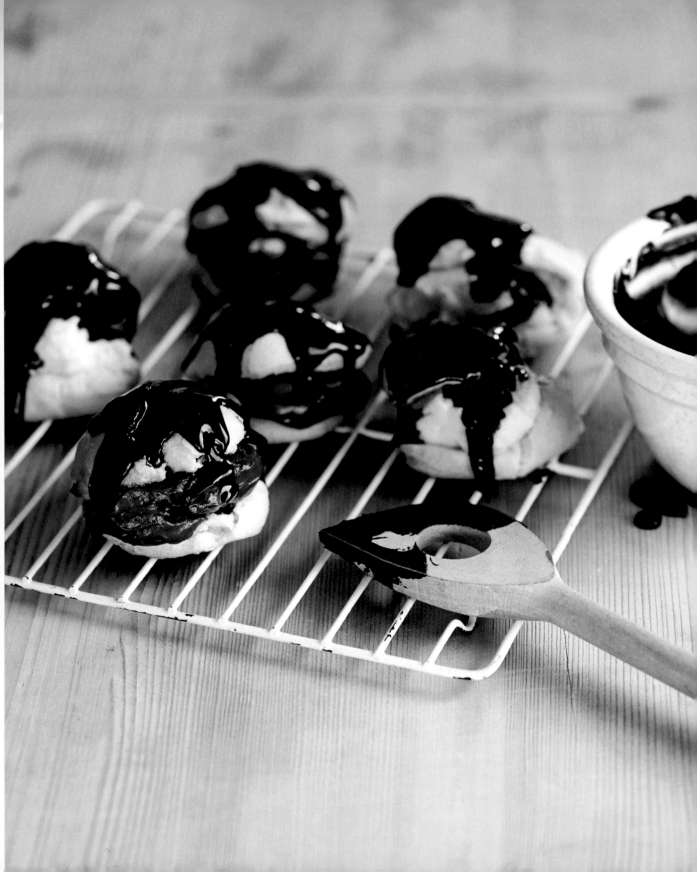

Cream Puffs with Chocolate Sauce

SERVES 6–8

Choux pastry, which is a feature ingredient in cream puffs, éclairs and other elegant desserts, may seem daunting, but it really couldn't be simpler. Just follow the steps and you'll be fine. I have suggested two different fillings in the recipe, but if you only want to make one, just double the quantities of one set of ingredients and omit the other.

1. Preheat the oven to 200°C. Line two baking sheets with parchment paper.

2. Combine the butter and 185 ml water in a medium saucepan and bring to a boil. Mix the rice flour and xanthan gum in a bowl until well combined, then add to the pan and beat quickly with a wooden spoon. The mixture will come away from the side of the pan and form a smooth ball.

3. Transfer the dough to a medium bowl. With a handheld electric mixer, beat in the sugar. Beat in the eggs one at a time.

4. Place rounded teaspoons of the dough on the sheets, about 4 cm apart. Bake for 7 minutes, or until the pastries puff up. Reduce the temperature to 180°C and bake for 10 minutes more or until crisp and lightly browned.

5. Reduce the temperature to 140°C and remove one sheet from the oven. Quickly and carefully cut a small opening in the side of each pastry. Return the sheet to the oven and repeat with the second sheet. Bake for 5 minutes, or until the pastries have dried out.

6. Remove from the oven and let cool to room temperature. Carefully cut the pastries open. Remove and discard the soft centres without crushing the pastry cases.

7. While the pastries are cooling, to make the crème custard, pour the milk into a small heavy-bottomed saucepan over medium heat and bring to just below a boil. Beat the egg yolks and

(recipe continues)

75 g unsalted butter

130 g superfine white rice flour

1 teaspoon xanthan gum or guar gum

1 heaped tablespoon sugar

3 large eggs

CRÈME CUSTARD

500 ml semi-skimmed milk, lactose-free milk or suitable plant-based milk

6 large egg yolks

110 g caster sugar

50 g cornflour

2 teaspoons vanilla extract

CHOCOLATE CUSTARD

50 g cornflour

625 ml semi-skimmed milk, lactose-free milk or suitable plant-based milk

3½ teaspoons sugar

115 g good-quality dark chocolate, broken into small pieces

2 tablespoons plus 2 teaspoons coffee liqueur or brewed strong espresso mixed with a bit of unsweetened cocoa powder

½ teaspoon vanilla extract

CHOCOLATE SAUCE

115 g good-quality dark chocolate, broken into pieces

80 ml single cream

Chocolate Soufflés

SERVES 6

A simple chocolate soufflé is hard to beat, but if you want to play around with the flavours a bit, add 1 heaped tablespoon instant coffee to the melted chocolate–cream mixture for a mocha flavour, or for chocolate-mint, replace the dark chocolate with gluten-free peppermint-filled chocolate.

Non-stick cooking spray

275 g caster sugar

225 g good-quality dark chocolate, broken into pieces

125 ml single cream

6 large eggs, separated

100 g cornflour

55 g light brown sugar

125 ml semi-skimmed milk, lactose-free milk or suitable plant-based milk

Icing sugar, sifted (optional)

1. Preheat the oven to 180°C.

2. Grease six 250-ml soufflé dishes with cooking spray. Place 1 tablespoon of the caster sugar in each dish and turn to coat generously, discarding any excess.

3. Combine the chocolate and cream in a heatproof bowl or the top part of a double boiler. Set over a saucepan of simmering water or the bottom part of the double boiler (make sure the bottom of the bowl does not touch the water) and stir until the chocolate is melted and well combined. Set aside to cool slightly.

4. Combine the egg yolks and remaining caster sugar in a large bowl and beat with a handheld electric mixer until pale, thick and creamy. Gradually beat in the cornflour, brown sugar and milk until combined. Pour into a saucepan and cook, stirring, over medium heat for 5 minutes, or until thickened. Stir into the chocolate mixture and set aside to cool slightly.

5. Clean the mixer beaters and beat the egg whites in a large clean bowl until stiff peaks form. Gently fold into the chocolate mixture with a large metal spoon, Fill the soufflé dishes to approximately 5 mm below the rim.

6. Place the dishes on a baking sheet and bake for 20 to 25 minutes, until the soufflés are nicely risen. Dust with icing sugar, if desired, and serve immediately, as they will sink if left standing.

PER SERVING (not including icing sugar): 544 calories; 10 g protein; 22 g total fat; 12 g saturated fat; 85 g carbohydrates; 3 g fibre; 89 mg sodium

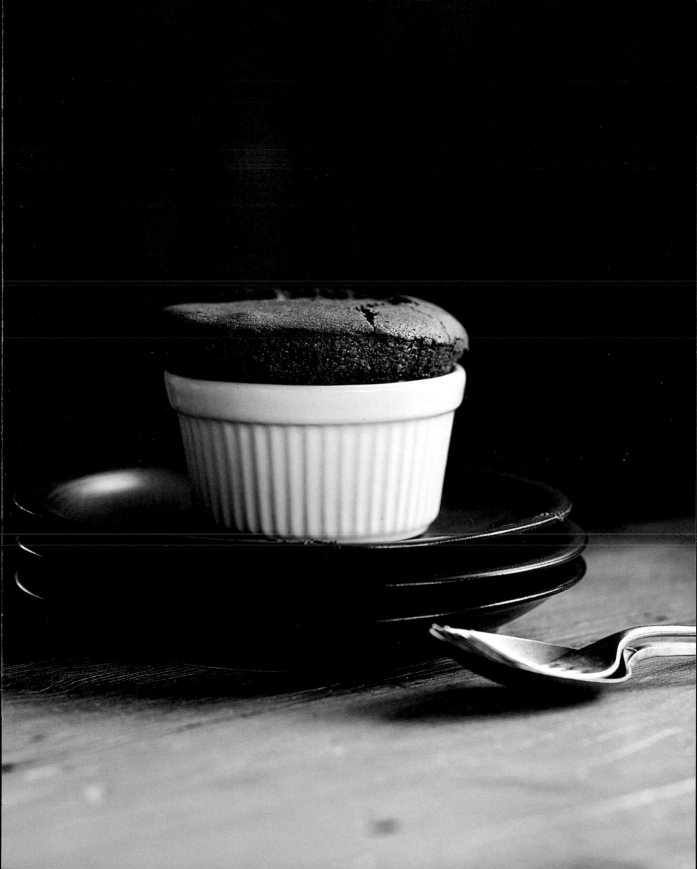

Irish Cream Delights

SERVES 6

I'm rather partial to the flavour of Irish cream liqueur, so I developed this recipe as a way to enjoy it in every mouthful of this smooth custard dessert.

125 ml single cream

110 g light brown sugar

500 ml milk, lactose-free milk or suitable plant-based milk

125 ml Irish cream liqueur, such as Baileys

35 g cornflour

Shaved chocolate, for serving

1. Combine the cream, brown sugar and 435 ml of the milk in a medium saucepan and cook over medium heat until almost boiling. Stir in the liqueur.

2. Blend the cornflour with the remaining 60 ml of milk to form a smooth paste. Gradually add to the warm cream mixture, stirring constantly to ensure there are no lumps, then cook, stirring, over medium heat for about 5 minutes, until thickened. (Don't let it boil.)

3. Pour the pudding into six 125-ml ramekins. Allow to cool, then cover with cling film and refrigerate for 3 to 4 hours, until set.

4. Decorate with the shaved chocolate just before serving.

PER SERVING (not including shaved chocolate): 230 calories; 4 g protein; 8 g total fat; 5 g saturated fat; 32 g carbohydrates; 0 g fibre; 76 mg sodium

---

NOTE: If you have lactose intolerance, this recipe is not suitable for you unless consumed in very small amounts. If you would like to enjoy a regular serving size, I recommend that you first take an adequate number of lactase enzyme tablets (available at pharmacies).

Berry and Chocolate Fudge Sundaes

SERVES 6–8

This recipe proves the notion that simple things are often the best – berries, chocolate and creamy vanilla ice cream. No fuss, just pure enjoyment – especially the rich chocolate fudge sauce.

1. To make the chocolate fudge sauce, melt the butter in a small saucepan over low heat. Add the brown sugar, cream, cocoa and dark chocolate and stir until the chocolate has melted and the sauce is smooth. Remove from the heat and let cool to room temperature.

2. Combine the berries in a bowl. Scoop the ice cream into serving glasses or bowls, scatter the berries on top and finish with a generous drizzle of chocolate fudge sauce.

PER SERVING (⅛ recipe): 302 calories; 4 g protein; 13 g total fat; 8 g saturated fat; 47 g carbohydrates; 4 g fibre; 60 mg sodium

CHOCOLATE FUDGE SAUCE

45 g unsalted butter

110 g light brown sugar

125 ml single cream

2 heaped tablespoons unsweetened cocoa powder

55 g good-quality dark chocolate buttons or chips

200 g blueberries

200 g raspberries

500 g strawberries, hulled, halved if large

1 litre gluten-free, lactose-free vanilla ice cream

Warm Lemon Tapioca Pudding

SERVES 6

Tapioca has made a comeback! This modern take on an old favourite is served warm and brings together a wonderfully creamy texture and a delicious tart lemon flavour.

4 lemons

1 litre semi-skimmed milk, lactose-free milk or suitable plant-based milk

100 g pearl tapioca or sago

75 g caster sugar

1. Using a vegetable peeler, slice the zest of all 4 lemons into 2-cm strips. Juice the lemons until you have 125 ml juice.

2. Combine the milk and lemon zest in a medium saucepan and bring to a simmer over high heat. Reduce the heat to low and simmer for 2 minutes. Remove and discard the lemon zest.

3. Add the tapioca to the milk, stirring well to combine. Simmer over low heat, stirring regularly, for 20 to 25 minutes, until the tapioca resembles translucent jellylike balls.

4. Remove from the heat. Stir in the sugar and lemon juice and pour into six glass dessert dishes. Serve immediately.

PER SERVING: 161 calories; 5 g protein; 2 g total fat; 1 g saturated fat; 32 g carbohydrates; 0 g fibre; 83 mg sodium

White Chocolate–Mint Pots

SERVES 4

While this dessert tastes decadent, it is actually a little less naughty than traditional chocolate mousse. The mint can be replaced with orange if you like, and you can use milk or dark chocolate instead of white to achieve a richer flavour. If you do this, omit the green colouring.

500 ml milk, lactose-free milk or suitable plant-based milk

60 ml single cream

110 g caster sugar

¼ teaspoon peppermint extract (more to taste)

3 or 4 drops green food colouring

115 g white chocolate chips, plus more for decorating

35 g cornflour

Mint leaves

1. Combine 185 ml of the milk and the cream, sugar, peppermint extract and food colouring in a small saucepan over medium heat and bring to just below a boil (don't let it boil). Add the white chocolate chips and stir until completely melted.

2. Blend the cornflour with the remaining 60 ml of milk to form a smooth paste. Gradually add to the white chocolate mixture, stirring constantly to ensure there are no lumps. Cook, stirring, for 5 minutes, or until thickened. Pour into four 200-ml ramekins. Allow to cool at room temperature, then refrigerate for 3 to 4 hours, until set.

3. Decorate with extra white chocolate chips and mint leaves just before serving.

PER SERVING: 372 calories; 6 g protein; 13 g total fat; 9 g saturated fat; 55 g carbohydrates; 0 g fibre; 100 mg sodium

---

NOTE: If you have lactose intolerance, this recipe is not suitable for you unless consumed in very small amounts. If you would like to enjoy a regular serving size, I recommend that you first take an adequate number of lactase enzyme tablets (available at pharmacies).

ICE CREAM, PUDDINGS & CUSTARDS

195

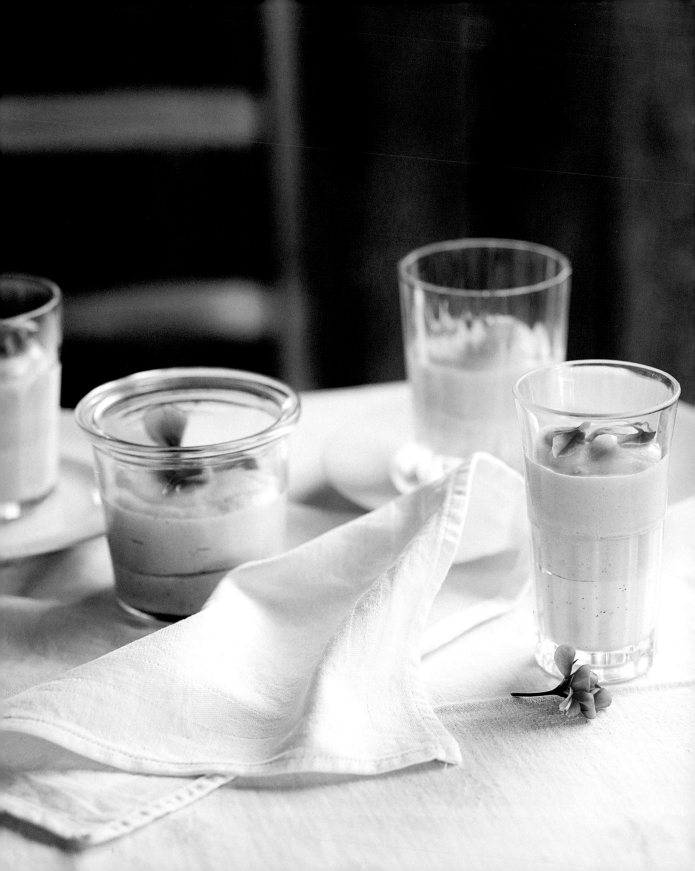

Cappuccino and Vanilla Bean Mousse Duo

SERVES 6

You can buy the dishes for this dessert in kitchenware and housewares stores, where you will find many different styles. Coffee cups work well, as do glasses, as we used in the photo. If you prefer, you can layer the mousses in a single larger dish and serve it in the centre of the table.

1. Grease six 150 ml glasses or ramekins with non-stick cooking spray.

2. Combine the chocolate and single cream in a heatproof bowl or the top part of a double boiler. Set over a saucepan of simmering water or the bottom part of the double boiler (make sure the bottom of the bowl does not touch the water) and stir until melted and well combined. Set aside to cool for 15 to 20 minutes.

3. Pour 125 ml cold water into a small heatproof bowl and whisk in the gelatin with a fork. Set aside for 5 minutes, or until the gelatin has softened. Fill a larger bowl with boiling water, set the bowl containing the gelatin in it and stir constantly until the gelatin has completely dissolved.

4. Stir the gelatin into the cooled chocolate mixture, then stir in the egg yolks, one at a time. Pour half of the chocolate mixture into another bowl.

5. Combine the whipping cream and sugar in a clean bowl and beat with a handheld electric mixer until the mixture is thick and the sugar has dissolved. Spoon half of the whipped cream into a smaller bowl.

6. Clean the mixer beaters. Beat the egg whites in a large clean bowl until stiff peaks form.

7. Add the vanilla to one of the bowls of chocolate mixture. With a large metal spoon, fold this into one of the bowls of

Non-stick cooking spray

225 g good-quality white chocolate, broken into pieces

150 ml single cream

1 heaped tablespoon unflavoured gelatin powder

4 large eggs, separated, at room temperature

250 ml whipping cream

55 g caster sugar

1 teaspoon vanilla bean paste or 1 to 2 teaspoons vanilla extract

2 teaspoons instant coffee

Edible organic flowers (optional)

(recipe continues)

whipped cream until well combined. Finally, gently fold in half of the beaten egg whites. Pour into the glasses. Cover and refrigerate for 1 hour, or until set. Let the other bowls sit at room temperature.

8. After an hour, dissolve the coffee in 2 tablespoons hot water and stir it into the remaining chocolate mixture. Fold this into the remaining whipped cream, then gently fold in the remaining egg whites. Pour into the glasses over the vanilla layer. Cover and refrigerate for 2 hours more or until set.

9. Just before serving, garnish with flowers, if desired.

PER SERVING: 470 calories; 9 g protein; 33 g total fat; 20 g saturated fat; 33 g carbohydrates; 0 g fibre; 108 mg sodium

---

NOTE: If you have lactose intolerance, this recipe is not suitable for you unless consumed in very small amounts. If you would like to enjoy a regular serving size, I recommend that you first take an adequate number of lactase enzyme tablets (available at pharmacies).

Cinnamon Panna Cotta with Puréed Banana

SERVES 4

This unusual dessert brings together the dynamic duo of banana and cinnamon. While the panna cotta can be made ahead, the banana purée should be prepared just before serving to prevent discolouration.

1. Grease four 125-ml dariole moulds, custard cups or tall ramekins with cooking spray.

2. Combine the cream, milk, caster sugar, cinnamon, and vanilla in a medium saucepan over low heat. Cook, stirring regularly, taking care not to let it boil, for 20 minutes, or until the mixture is thick enough to coat the back of a spoon. Remove from the heat and pour into a medium heatproof bowl.

3. Add 1 tablespoon of cold water to a small heatproof bowl and whisk in the gelatin with a fork. Set it aside for 5 minutes, or until the gelatin has begun to gel. Fill a larger bowl with boiling water, set the bowl containing the gelatin in it, and stir constantly until the gelatin has completely dissolved. Whisk into the cream mixture.

4. Fill a large bowl with ice cubes. Place the bowl with the cream mixture on the ice and whisk every few minutes for about 10 minutes. The mixture will thicken as it cools. When it is thick enough to coat the back of a spoon, carefully pour it into the moulds. Refrigerate, covered, for 2 to 3 hours, until set.

5. Combine the bananas and brown sugar in a bowl and mash with a fork until smooth and well combined.

6. To serve, dip each mould in hot water for a few seconds, then turn out onto plates. Spoon the puréed banana into a piping bag and use to decorate the plates (or dollop directly onto the panna cotta, if preferred).

PER SERVING: 370 calories; 5 g protein; 20 g total fat; 12 g saturated fat; 46 g carbohydrates; 2 g fibre; 60 mg sodium

Non-stick cooking spray

420 ml single cream

125 ml milk, lactose-free milk or suitable plant-based milk

110 g caster sugar

1 teaspoon ground cinnamon

1 teaspoon vanilla extract

2¼ teaspoons unflavoured gelatin powder

Ice cubes

2 ripe bananas, peeled

2 teaspoons light brown sugar

NOTE: If you have lactose intolerance, this recipe is not suitable for you unless consumed in very small amounts. If you would like to enjoy a regular serving size, I recommend that you first take an adequate number of lactase enzyme tablets (available at pharmacies).

ICE CREAM, PUDDINGS & CUSTARDS

Orange-Scented Panna Cotta

Panna cotta literally means 'cooked cream'. This lighter version of the traditional Italian dessert features a delicate hint of orange.

1. Grease four 125-ml dariole moulds, custard cups or tall ramekins with cooking spray.

2. To make the topping, combine all the ingredients in a small heatproof bowl. Set the bowl over a larger bowl of boiling water and stir until the gelatin has completely dissolved.

3. Pour one quarter of the orange topping into each cup. Refrigerate for 1 to 2 hours, until set.

4. Combine the cream, milk, caster sugar, orange zest and orange juice in a medium saucepan over low heat. Cook, stirring regularly, taking care not to let it boil, for 20 minutes, or until it has thickened enough to coat the back of a spoon. Remove from the heat and pour into a medium heatproof bowl.

5. Pour 1 tablespoon cold water into a small heatproof bowl and whisk in the gelatin with a fork. Set it aside for 5 minutes, or until the gelatin has begun to gel. Fill a larger bowl with boiling water, set the bowl containing the gelatin in it and stir constantly until the gelatin has completely dissolved. Whisk into the cream mixture.

6. Fill another large bowl with ice cubes. Place the bowl with the cream mixture on the ice and whisk every few minutes for about 10 minutes. The mixture will thicken as it cools. When it is thick enough to coat the back of a spoon, carefully pour it over the orange topping in the moulds. Refrigerate, covered, for 2 to 3 hours, until set.

7. To serve, dip mould in hot water for a few seconds, then turn out onto plates. Serve garnished with fresh orange segments.

PER SERVING: 359 calories; 6 g protein; 20 g total fat; 12 g saturated fat; 42 g carbohydrates; 1 g fibre; 62 mg sodium

Non-stick cooking spray

ORANGE TOPPING

2 tablespoons plus 2 teaspoons fresh orange juice, strained

2 tablespoons plus 2 teaspoons boiling water

2 tablespoons plus 2 teaspoons sugar

1½ teaspoons unflavoured gelatin powder

420 ml single cream

125 ml milk, lactose-free milk or suitable plant-based milk

110 g caster sugar

3 to 4 heaped tablespoons finely grated orange zest

2 tablespoons plus 2 teaspoons fresh orange juice, strained

2¼ teaspoons unflavoured gelatin powder

Ice cubes

Orange segments, for serving

NOTE: If you have lactose intolerance, this recipe is not suitable for you unless consumed in very small amounts. If you would like to enjoy a regular serving size, I recommend that you first take an adequate number of lactase enzyme tablets (available at pharmacies).

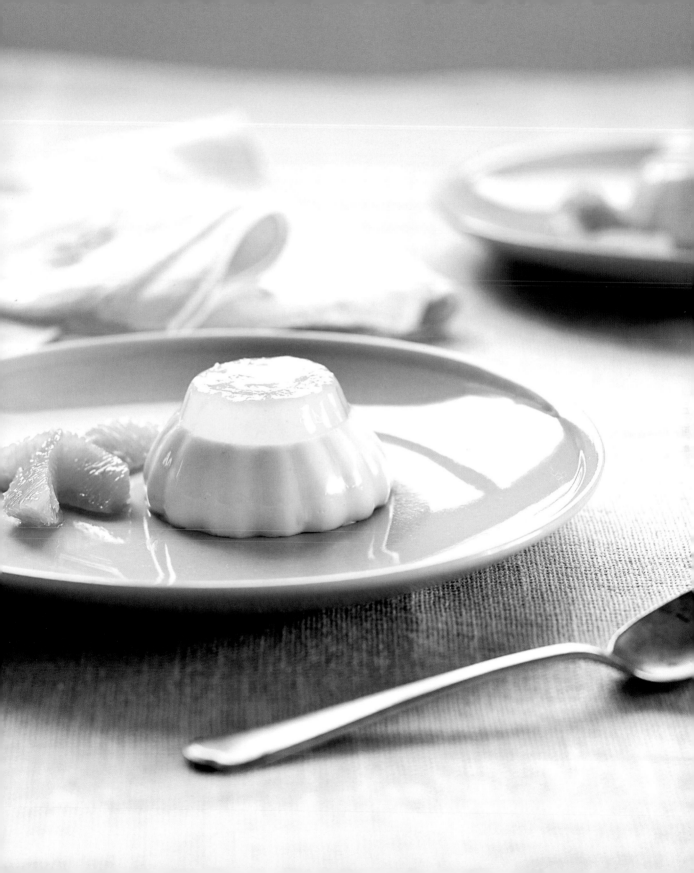

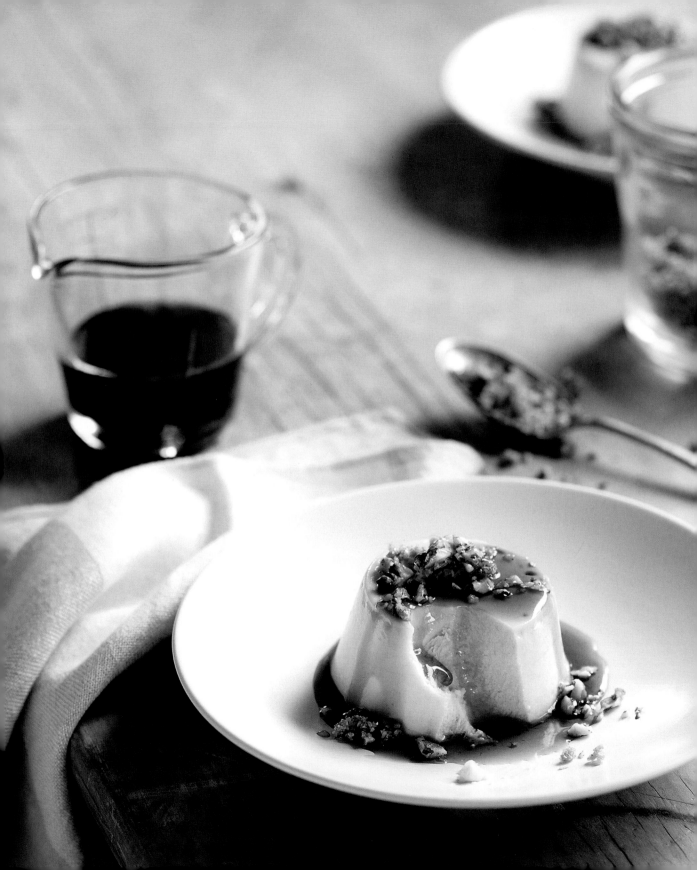

Maple Syrup Bavarian Cream with Quick Pecan Brittle

SERVES 6

Unlike honey, maple syrup is suitable for people on a low-FODMAP diet because the fructose content is balanced by glucose. This is great news, because its distinctive flavour is widely beloved. Coupled with buttery pecans, it makes this dessert taste as good as it looks!

1. Grease six 125-ml dariole moulds, custard cups or tall ramekins with cooking spray.

2. Place the egg yolks and sugar in a medium bowl and beat with a handheld electric mixer for 2 to 3 minutes, until thick and pale.

3. Combine the maple syrup and milk in a medium saucepan over low heat. Whisk in the egg mixture and stir with a wooden spoon over very low heat for 5 minutes, or until thick enough to coat the back of the spoon. Don't let it boil. Remove from the heat and pour into a medium heatproof bowl.

4. Add 3 tablespoons of cold water to a small heatproof bowl and whisk in the gelatin with a fork. Set it aside for 5 minutes, or until the gelatin has begun to gel. Fill a larger bowl with boiling water, set the bowl containing the gelatin in it and stir constantly until the gelatin has completely dissolved. Whisk the gelatin into the maple mixture until smooth.

5. Fill a large bowl with ice cubes. Place the bowl with the maple mixture on the ice and whisk every few minutes for about 10 minutes. The mixture will thicken as it cools.

6. Beat the cream in a medium bowl with a handheld electric mixer until thick. Fold into the cooled maple mixture with a large metal spoon until well combined. Pour evenly into the moulds, then place the moulds on a baking sheet, cover with cling film, and refrigerate for 4 to 5 hours.

(recipe continues)

Non-stick cooking spray

3 large egg yolks, at room temperature

110 g caster sugar

125 ml maple syrup

125 ml semi-skimmed milk, lactose-free milk or suitable plant-based milk

1 heaped tablespoon unflavoured gelatin powder

Ice cubes

250 ml whipping cream

QUICK PECAN BRITTLE

50 g gluten-free butterscotch sweets

60 g pecans, coarsely crushed

7. To make the pecan brittle, combine the butterscotch and pecans in a small food processor or blender and process until coarsely crushed (don't overdo it or you will be left with crumbs).

8. To serve, dip each mould into hot water for a few seconds, then turn out onto plates. Sprinkle generously with the pecan brittle.

PER SERVING: 391 calories; 5 g protein; 23 g total fat; 9 g saturated fat; 45 g carbohydrates; 1 g fibre; 62 mg sodium

---

NOTE: If you have lactose intolerance, this recipe is not suitable for you unless consumed in very small amounts. If you would like to enjoy a regular serving size, I recommend that you first take an adequate number of lactase enzyme tablets (available at pharmacies).

Lemon Tart

SERVES 8–10

This luscious tart has become a favourite at our family get-togethers. Everyone in my family knows by heart how to make it, and I hope that before long, you will, too!

1. Preheat the oven to 180°C. Grease a 23-cm fluted tart tin with cooking spray.

2. To make the pastry, sift the rice flour, cornflour, soy flour and xanthan gum into a bowl. Transfer to a food processor, add the caster sugar and butter, and process until the mixture resembles fine breadcrumbs. While the motor is running, add the ice water (a tablespoon at a time) to form a soft dough.

3. Lightly sprinkle your work surface with cornflour. Turn out the dough onto the work surface and knead until smooth. Wrap in cling film and refrigerate for 30 minutes.

4. Place the dough between two sheets of parchment paper and roll out to a thickness of about 2 to 3 mm. Ease the pastry into the tin and trim the edges to neaten.

5. Line the pastry with parchment paper, fill with baking beans or rice and bake for 10 minutes, or until lightly golden. Remove the beans and parchment. Reduce the oven temperature to 160°C.

6. To make the filling, combine the caster sugar, mascarpone, lemon zest and lemon juice in a medium bowl and beat with a handheld electric mixer. Add the eggs one at a time, beating well between additions. Pour the filling into the warm pastry case and bake for 30 to 35 minutes, until set.

7. Cool completely in the tin. Dust with icing sugar before serving.

PER SERVING (1/10 recipe): 408 calories; 8 g protein; 24 g total fat; 8 g saturated fat; 42 g carbohydrates; 1 g fibre; 50 mg sodium

Non-stick cooking spray

PASTRY

130 g superfine white rice flour

75 g cornflour, plus more for kneading

45 g soy flour

1 teaspoon xanthan gum or guar gum

55 g caster sugar

150 g cold unsalted butter, diced

About 100–125 ml ice water

165 g caster sugar

225 g packet mascarpone

1 heaped tablespoon finely grated lemon zest

165 ml fresh lemon juice

4 large eggs

Icing sugar, for dusting

Citrus Rice Tart with Raspberry Sauce

SERVES 8–10

This is rice pudding with a big twist! Combined with the fabulous flavours of orange and lemon, it sets firm into a tart. Serve it with a generous drizzle of the vibrant raspberry sauce.

1. Preheat the oven to 160°C. Grease a 23-cm fluted tart or pie tin with cooking spray.

2. Bring 1.5 litres water to a boil in a large saucepan. Add the rice and sugar and cook, stirring occasionally, for 12 minutes, or until the rice is tender. Drain and rinse under cold water to cool.

3. Combine the cornflour, eggs, cream, vanilla, orange zest and juice and lemon zest in a medium bowl. Add the rice and mix well. Pour into the tart tin and bake for 35 to 40 minutes, until just set.

4. Remove from the oven and let cool to room temperature, then refrigerate for 2 to 3 hours.

5. Remove from the refrigerator 30 minutes before serving. If your tin has a removable bottom, slip off the outer rim.

6. To make the raspberry sauce, blend all the ingredients in a blender or food processor. Serve drizzled over the tart.

PER SERVING (1/10 recipe): 234 calories; 4 g protein; 4 g total fat; 2 g saturated fat; 45 g carbohydrates; 1 g fibre; 37 mg sodium

---

NOTE: If you have trouble finding tinned raspberries, combine 185 g fresh or frozen raspberries with 55 g icing sugar. Cover and refrigerate until juicy and syrupy, about 1 hour, then follow step 6.

Non-stick cooking spray

200 g medium-grain white rice

55 g sugar

50 g cornflour

3 large eggs

150 ml single cream

½ teaspoon vanilla extract

Grated zest of 1 orange

180 ml fresh orange juice

Grated zest of 1 lemon

RASPBERRY SAUCE

One 425-g tin raspberries in syrup, drained, reserving the juice (see Note)

60 ml raspberry juice (from the tin)

1 heaped tablespoon icing sugar

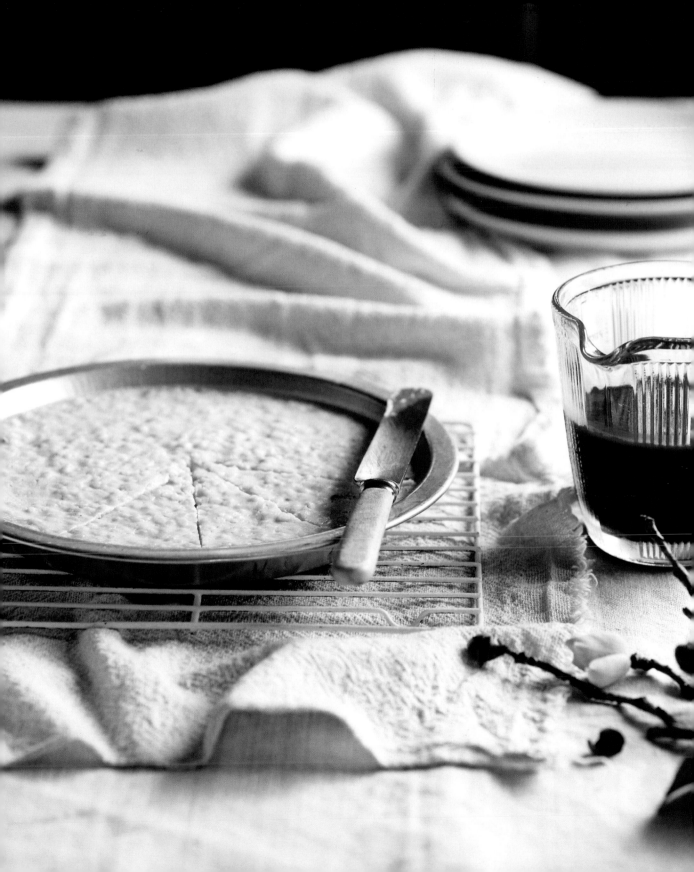

Lemon Tartlets

MAKES 12

If you don't have time to make your own pastry, you can purchase ready-made pastry shells from the freezer section of larger supermarkets and health food shops.

1. Preheat the oven to 170°C. Grease twelve tartlet tins or a 12-cup muffin tin with cooking spray.

2. To make the filling, blend the cornflour with 1 tablespoon of the water in a small saucepan to form a smooth paste. Add the remaining water, stirring to ensure there are no lumps, then add the lemon zest, lemon juice, butter and sugar and stir over medium-low heat until thickened, 3 to 5 minutes. Remove from the heat and let cool for 10 minutes. Stir in the egg yolks. Pour into a bowl, cover and refrigerate until cold.

3. Meanwhile, place the chilled dough between two sheets of parchment paper and roll out to a thickness of about 2 to 3 mm. Cut out 12 rounds with a pastry cutter to fit the tin or cups. Place in the tin or cups and trim the edges to neaten. Bake for 12 to 15 minutes, until golden. Let cool on a wire rack.

4. Spoon the chilled lemon filling into the tartlet cases and serve with ice cream.

PER SERVING: 297 calories; 4 g protein; 15 g total fat; 9 g saturated fat; 39 g carbohydrates; 1 g fibre; 12 mg sodium

Non-stick cooking spray

LEMON FILLING

75 g cornflour

300 ml water

Grated zest of 2 lemons

180 ml fresh lemon juice

60 g unsalted butter, cut into cubes, at room temperature

150 g sugar

2 large egg yolks

1 batch Pastry dough, chilled (page 205)

Gluten-free, lactose-free ice cream, for serving

Cinnamon and Chestnut Flan

SERVES 10–12

Chestnut meal (not to be confused with chestnut flour) is crushed chestnuts, and has a grainy, mealy texture. It may be available from gourmet food stores or online and should be stored in the freezer or fridge. If you can't find it, substitute puréed chestnuts (either tinned or homemade; see the head-note on page 84).

Non-stick cooking spray

1 batch Pastry dough (page 205), chilled

165 g caster sugar

2 tablespoons ground cinnamon

One 396-g tin fat-free sweetened condensed milk

One 225-g packet mascarpone or reduced-fat cream cheese, at room temperature

225 g chestnut meal

4 large eggs

Icing sugar, for dusting

Gluten-free, lactose-free ice cream, for serving

1. Preheat the oven to 170°C. Grease a 23-cm fluted quiche tin with cooking spray.

2. Place the chilled dough between two sheets of parchment paper and roll out to a thickness of about 2 to 3 mm. Ease the pastry into the flan dish and trim the edges to neaten.

3. Line the pastry with parchment paper, fill with baking beans or rice, and bake for 10 minutes, or until lightly golden. Remove from the oven and reduce the oven temperature to 160°C. Remove the beans and parchment.

4. Meanwhile, to make the filling, combine the caster sugar, cinnamon, condensed milk, mascarpone, chestnut meal and eggs in a food processor or blender and blend until smooth and well combined. Pour the filling into the warm pastry case.

5. Bake for 50 to 60 minutes, until set. Remove and let cool completely in the tin before serving.

6. Dust with icing sugar and serve with ice cream.

PER SERVING (1/12 recipe): 506 calories; 8 g protein; 21 g total fat; 7 g saturated fat; 71 g carbohydrates; 3 g fibre; 188 mg sodium

Lemon Cheesecake

SERVES 10–12

This cheesecake has a sweet, zesty topping, which gives a lovely fresh contrast to the creamy filling. If you prefer to keep things simple, however, leave off the topping.

1. Mix together the crushed biscuits and melted butter in a medium bowl. Press evenly into the bottom of a 20-cm springform tin. Refrigerate while you prepare the filling and topping.

2. To make the filling, add 125 ml cold water to a small heat-proof bowl and whisk in the gelatin with a fork. Set aside for 5 minutes, or until the gelatin has begun to gel. Fill a larger bowl with boiling water, set the bowl containing the gelatin into it and stir constantly until the gelatin has completely dissolved.

3. Combine the cream cheese, sugar, lemon juice, lemon zest and dissolved gelatin in a food processor or blender and process for 1 to 2 minutes, until smooth.

4. Beat the cream in a medium bowl with a handheld electric mixer until thickened. Using a large metal spoon, fold the whipped cream into the cream cheese mixture. Pour the filling onto the biscuit base. Cover and refrigerate for 3 hours, until set.

5. To make the topping, add 125 ml cold water to a small heat-proof bowl and whisk in the gelatin with a fork. Set aside for 5 minutes, until the gelatin has begun to gel. Fill a larger bowl with boiling water, set the bowl containing the gelatin in it and stir constantly until the gelatin has completely dissolved.

6. Combine the dissolved gelatin, butter, sugar, egg yolk and lemon zest and juice in a small saucepan. Stir over low heat for about 15 minutes, until thick enough to coat the back of a spoon. Let cool to room temperature.

7. Pour the topping evenly over the filling, then return the cheesecake to the refrigerator for at least 3 hours, until set.

PER SERVING (1/12 recipe): 380 calories; 7 g protein; 24 g total fat; 12 g saturated fat; 37 g carbohydrates; 1 g fibre; 160 mg sodium

250 g gluten-free vanilla biscuits, crushed

60 g unsalted butter, melted

CHEESECAKE FILLING

1 heaped tablespoon unflavoured gelatin powder

One 225-g packet reduced-fat cream cheese, at room temperature

165 g caster sugar

2 tablespoons plus 2 teaspoons fresh lemon juice

1 to 2 heaped tablespoons grated lemon zest

300 ml whipping cream

LEMON TOPPING

1½ teaspoons unflavoured gelatin powder

45 g unsalted butter, cut into cubes, at room temperature

110 g caster sugar

1 large egg yolk, lightly beaten

1 teaspoon grated lemon zest

2 tablespoons plus 2 teaspoons fresh lemon juice

NOTE: If you have lactose intolerance, this recipe is not suitable unless consumed in very small amounts. If you would like to enjoy a regular serving size, first take an adequate number of lactase enzyme tablets.

Baked Blueberry Cheesecakes

SERVES 9

Making these in miniature allows each guest to have an individual serving. However, you certainly can make this into one big cheesecake if you prefer. Use a 23-cm springform tin if you wish to do this, and bake, covered, for 50 to 60 minutes.

1. Preheat the oven to 160°C.

2. Mix together the crushed biscuits and melted butter, then press into the bottom of nine 10-cm springform tins. Divide the blueberries evenly over the biscuit bases.

3. Combine the cream cheese, condensed milk, vanilla, cream, eggs and cornflour in a food processor or blender and process until smooth. Pour the batter over the bases. Bake for 15 to 20 minutes, until lightly golden and firm to the touch.

4. Allow to cool completely in the tins, then cover and refrigerate for 3 hours before serving.

PER SERVING: 512 calories; 9 g protein; 18 g total fat; 9 g saturated fat; 37 g carbohydrates; 1 g fibre; 252 mg sodium

---

NOTE: If you have lactose intolerance, this recipe is not suitable for you unless consumed in very small amounts. If you would like to enjoy a regular serving size, I recommend that you first take an adequate number of lactase enzyme tablets (available at pharmacies).

250 g gluten-free vanilla biscuits, crushed

60 g unsalted butter, melted

300 g fresh or frozen blueberries

Two 225-g packets reduced-fat cream cheese, at room temperature

One 396-g tin fat-free sweetened condensed milk

2 teaspoons vanilla extract

125 ml whipping cream

2 large eggs

35 g cornflour

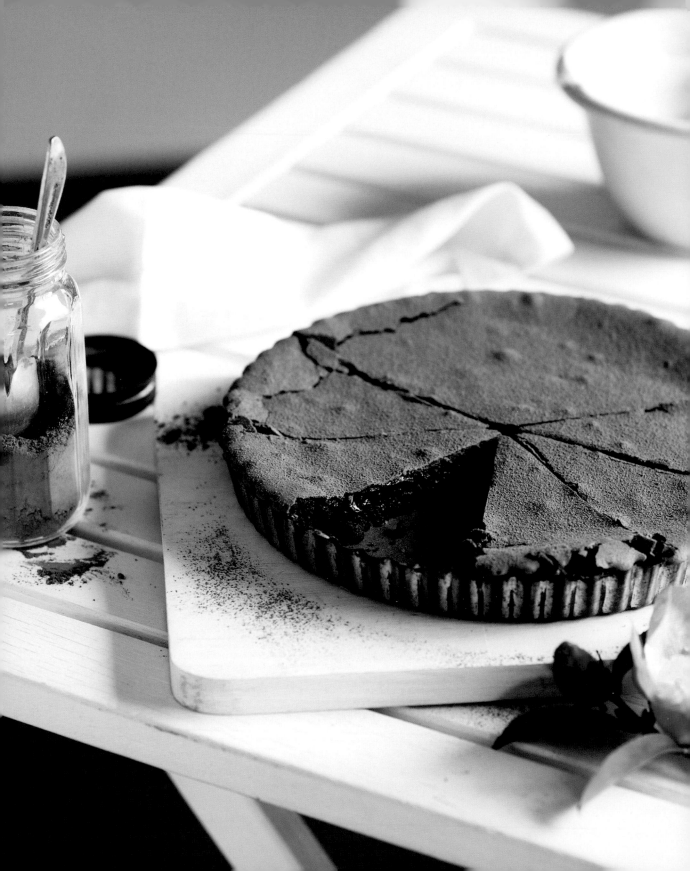

Chocolate Tart

This indulgent tart is very rich, so you only need a small serving – though you can always go back for seconds, and thirds! If gluten-free chocolate biscuits are unavailable, the tart can be made without a base. In this case, bake it in a greased 19-cm springform tin.

Non-stick cooking spray

200 g gluten-free chocolate biscuits, crushed

75 g unsalted butter, melted

CHOCOLATE FILLING

225 g good-quality dark chocolate, broken into pieces

150 g unsalted butter, cut into cubes, at room temperature

165 g caster sugar

2 teaspoons vanilla extract

60 ml coffee liqueur (optional)

5 large eggs, at room temperature

Unsweetened cocoa powder, for dusting

Gluten-free, lactose-free, ice cream, for serving

1. Preheat the oven to 150°C. Grease a 23-cm fluted tart tin with cooking spray.

2. Mix together the crushed biscuits and melted butter in a medium bowl. Press evenly into the bottom of the tart tin. Refrigerate while you prepare the filling.

3. To make the filling, place the chocolate in a small heatproof bowl or the top part of a double boiler. Set over a saucepan of simmering water or the bottom part of the double boiler (make sure the bottom of the bowl does not touch the water), stirring occasionally until melted. Set aside to cool slightly.

4. Combine the butter, sugar, vanilla, coffee liqueur (if using) and 1 egg in a medium bowl and beat with a handheld electric mixer until pale and creamy. Add the melted chocolate and beat until well combined. Set aside.

5. Clean the mixer beaters. Beat the remaining eggs in a large bowl for 3 to 5 minutes, until increased in volume by two or three times. Pour the chocolate mixture into the eggs and beat on low speed for 1 to 2 minutes, until combined.

6. Pour the filling evenly over the biscuit base and bake for 45 to 50 minutes, until set. Remove and let cool to room temperature, then refrigerate for 2 to 3 hours. Dust generously with cocoa and serve with ice cream.

PER SERVING (1/12 recipe, not including ice cream): 405 calories; 4 g protein; 26 g total fat; 15 g saturated fat; 36 g carbohydrates; 2 g fibre; 51 mg sodium

TARTS & CAKES

Pecan and Maple Tarts

MAKES 24

These are just the thing for people on a low-FODMAP diet to make as an alternative to apple pie during the festive season. Having said that, they are of course delicious all year round! The recipe can be halved for a smaller get-together.

1. Preheat the oven to 170°C. Grease two 12-cup mini tartlet or mini muffin tins with cooking spray. Line a baking sheet with parchment paper.

2. Place the chilled pastry dough between two sheets of parchment paper and roll out to a thickness of about 2 to 3 mm. Cut out 24 round crusts with a scalloped 3 to 4 cm pastry cutter to fit the mini tartlet tins. Place in the cups and trim the edges to neaten. Using a star-shaped cookie cutter (or other desired shape), cut out 24 small stars. Place the stars on the baking sheet. Bake the crusts and stars until golden (the crusts will take about 10 minutes, but the stars will only need 7 to 8 minutes). Remove from the oven and cool on a wire rack.

3. Increase the oven temperature to 180°C.

4. To make the filling, combine the butter, brown sugar and vanilla in a small bowl and beat with a handheld electric mixer until creamy. Beat in the egg and maple syrup, then stir in the chopped pecans.

5. Pour the filling evenly into the crusts and bake for 5 to 10 minutes, until the filling is set (it should remain firm when given a gentle shake). Place a star on each tart while still warm.

6. Cool in the pans for 10 minutes before removing and cooling completely on a wire rack. Dust with icing sugar, if desired.

PER SERVING: 218 calories; 4 g protein; 12 g total fat; 7 g saturated fat; 24 g carbohydrates; 1 g fibre; 114 mg sodium

Non-stick cooking spray

2 batches Pastry dough, chilled (page 205)

FILLING

15 g unsalted butter, at room temperature

55 g light brown sugar

½ teaspoon vanilla extract

1 large egg

60 ml maple syrup

60 g pecans, roughly chopped

icing sugar, for dusting (optional)

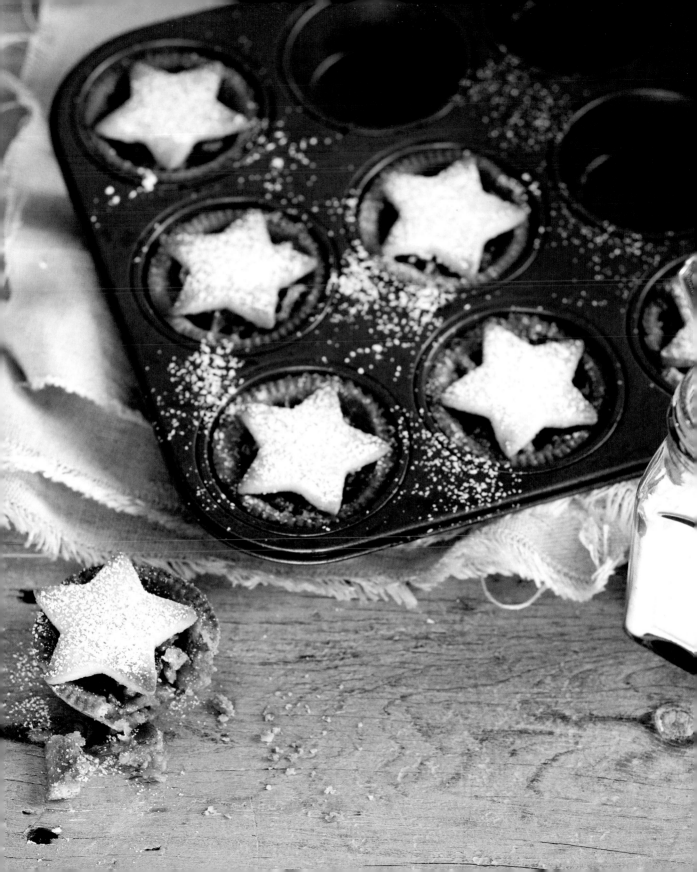

Layered Tahitian Lime Cheesecake

SERVES 10–12

I love the look of this cheesecake, and it is not difficult to make. The lime gives it a nice point of difference, but if you would rather use lemon instead, please feel free.

1. Mix together the crushed biscuits and melted butter in a medium bowl. Press evenly into the bottom of a 23-cm spring-form tin. Place in the refrigerator while you prepare the topping.

2. Add 125 ml cold water to a small heatproof bowl and whisk in the gelatin with a fork. Set aside for 5 minutes, or until the gelatin has begun to gel. Fill a larger bowl with boiling water, set the bowl containing the gelatin in it and stir constantly until the gelatin has completely dissolved.

3. Combine the dissolved gelatin, cream cheese and condensed milk in a food processor or blender and process for 1 minute, or until smooth.

4. Pour half of the mixture into a clean bowl; there should be about 500 ml. Add the coconut liqueur to the bowl and mix it in well. Pour over the biscuit base and freeze for 10 minutes.

5. Add the lime juice, lime zest and food colouring to the remaining batter in the food processor and process for 30 seconds, or until well combined.

6. Remove the cheesecake from the freezer – it should be just set. Pour the lime mixture over the coconut layer, then refrigerate for 2 to 3 hours to set completely before serving.

PER SERVING (¹⁄₁₂ **recipe**): 347 calories; 9 g protein; 16 g total fat; 8 g saturated fat; 39 g carbohydrates; 1 g fibre; 271 mg sodium

250 g gluten-free vanilla biscuits, crushed

60 g butter, melted

2 tablespoons unflavoured gelatin powder

Two 225-g packets reduced-fat cream cheese, at room temperature

One 396-g tin fat free sweetened condensed milk

80 ml coconut liqueur (see Notes)

3 tablespoons plus 1 teaspoon fresh lime juice

Finely grated zest of 1 lime

1 to 2 drops green food colouring

NOTES: If you have lactose intolerance, this recipe is not suitable for you unless consumed in very small amounts. If you would like to enjoy a regular serving size, I recommend that you first take an adequate number of lactase enzyme tablets (available at pharmacies). If you avoid alcohol, you may substitute 125 ml of coconut milk for the 80 ml of coconut liqueur, and add an extra ¼ teaspoon of gelatin powder.

Orange and Poppy Seed Cake

SERVES 10

There is not one person who has tried this cake who does not adore it. I have even been asked to ship a batch of it to an ill friend who was craving it! It did her the world of good, and whether or not you're currently feeling unwell, I think you'll enjoy it, too.

1. Preheat the oven to 170°C. Grease a 23-cm springform tin with cooking spray and line with a parchment paper circle.
2. Place the oranges in a medium saucepan of boiling water and boil, covered, for 20 minutes. Drain. Place the softened oranges in a food processor or blender and process (seeds, pith, and all!) for 3 to 4 minutes to form a smooth paste. Set aside to cool.
3. Sift the almond flour, baking powder and rice flour three times into a bowl (or whisk in the bowl until well combined). Stir in the poppy seeds.
4. Beat the eggs in a medium bowl with a handheld electric mixer for 5 minutes, or until thick and creamy. Add the sugar and beat until well combined.
5. Stir the orange paste into the dry ingredients, then fold into the egg mixture with a large metal spoon. Pour the batter into the pan and bake for 50 to 60 minutes, until golden brown and firm to the touch (a toothpick inserted into the centre should come out clean).
6. Cool in the pan for 15 minutes, then remove the outer ring and turn out onto a wire rack to cool completely.

PER SERVING: 355 calories; 11 g protein; 19 g total fat; 2 g saturated fat; 43 g carbohydrates; 5 g fibre; 80 mg sodium

Non-stick cooking spray

2 oranges

150 g almond flour

1 teaspoon gluten-free baking powder

65 g superfine white rice flour

2 tablespoons poppy seeds

5 large eggs

275 g sugar

Rich White Chocolate Cake

SERVES 12

I have to say upfront that this cake is super rich and super decadent. You may choose to top it with icing; however I don't usually – a dusting of icing sugar is really all it needs.

1. Preheat the oven to 150°C. Grease a 23-cm springform tin with cooking spray.

2. Combine the butter, white chocolate, brown sugar and 375 ml hot water in a medium heatproof bowl or the top part of a double boiler. Set over a saucepan of simmering water or the bottom part of the double boiler (make sure the bottom of the bowl does not touch the water) and stir until the chocolate and butter are melted and everything is well combined. Set aside to cool to room temperature.

3. Sift the soy flour, tapioca flour, rice flour, cornflour, xanthan gum, baking soda and baking powder three times into a medium bowl (or whisk in the bowl until well combined). Add the cooled white chocolate mixture, vanilla and eggs and beat with a hand-held electric mixer until smooth.

4. Pour the batter into the tin and bake for 45 minutes. Cover with foil and bake for 15 to 30 minutes more, until firm to the touch (a toothpick inserted into the centre should come out clean).

5. Cool in the pan for 15 minutes, then remove the outer ring and turn out onto a wire rack to cool completely. Dust with icing sugar before serving.

PER SERVING: 496 calories; 7 g protein; 21 g total fat; 13 g saturated fat; 73 g carbohydrates; 1 g fibre; 196 mg sodium

Non-stick cooking spray

225 g unsalted butter, cut into cubes

200 g good-quality white chocolate, broken into pieces

475 g light brown sugar

65 g soy flour

95 g tapioca flour

130 g superfine white rice flour

75 g cornflour

2 teaspoons xanthan gum or guar gum

1 teaspoon baking soda

1 teaspoon gluten-free baking powder

2 teaspoons vanilla extract

2 large eggs

Icing sugar, for dusting

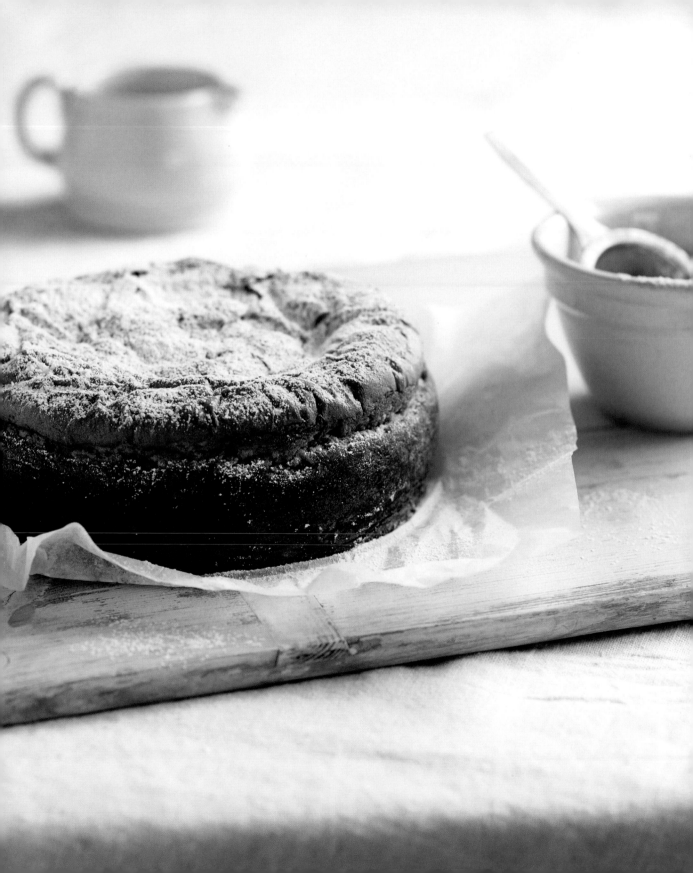

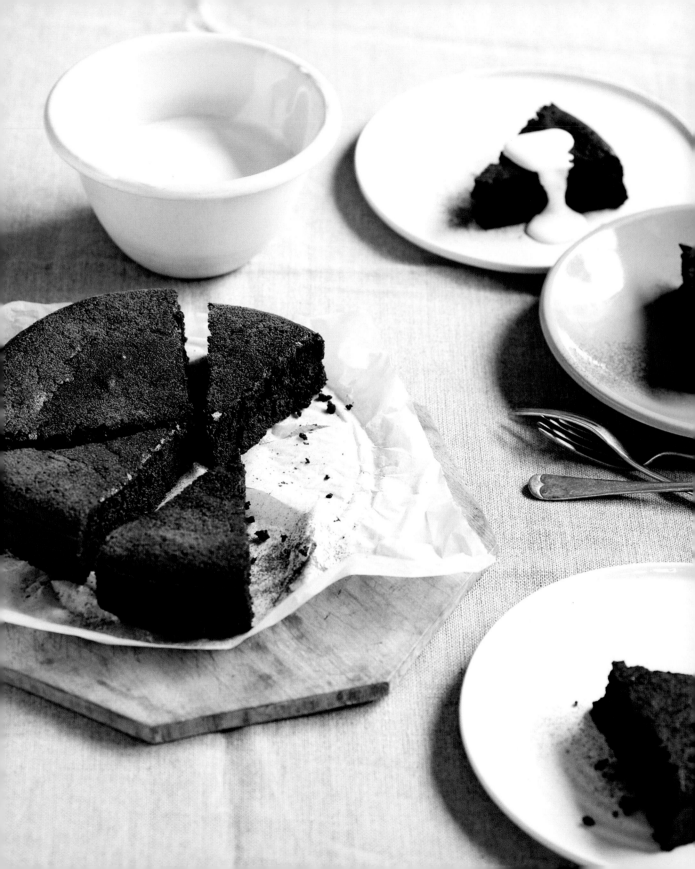

Flourless Chocolate Cake

Decadent and divine, this is the perfect dessert when you are entertaining. Serve it with ice cream (lactose-free, if necessary) and watch your guests savour every mouthful.

1. Preheat the oven to 150°C. Grease a 23-cm springform tin with cooking spray and line with a parchment paper circle.

2. Combine the cocoa, butter, dark chocolate and 80 ml water in a medium saucepan over low heat and stir until melted and smooth. Remove from the heat and stir in the brown sugar, almond flour and egg yolks. Transfer to a large bowl and let cool to room temperature.

3. Beat the egg whites in a clean bowl with a handheld electric mixer until soft peaks form. Gently fold the egg whites into the cooled chocolate mixture in two batches.

4. Pour the batter into the prepared springform tin and bake for 55 to 65 minutes, until firm when pressed gently in the centre.

5. Cool in the tin for 20 minutes, then remove the outer ring and turn out onto a wire rack to cool completely. Dust with additional cocoa and serve with ice cream, if desired.

PER SERVING (1/10 recipe, not including ice cream): 398 calories; 7 g protein; 26 g total fat; 12 g saturated fat; 40 g carbohydrates; 4 g fibre; 44 mg sodium

Non-stick cooking spray

35 g unsweetened cocoa powder, plus more for dusting

150 g unsalted butter, cut into cubes, at room temperature

150 g good-quality dark chocolate, broken into pieces

275 g light brown sugar

150 g almond flour

4 large eggs, separated

Gluten-free, lactose-free ice cream, for serving (optional)

Moist Chocolate Cake

SERVES 10–12

I figure every cookbook has to have at least one really great chocolate cake in it, and I get a lot of requests for this particular recipe. If you already own *The Complete Low-FODMAP Diet*, you'll notice this is similar to the Basic Chocolate Cake recipe that appears there – with a chocolate buttercream icing added on. This recipe is foolproof and delicious without any adornment, but it's also pretty special with the chocolate icing.

1. Preheat the oven to 170°C. Grease a 23-cm springform tin with cooking spray and line with a parchment paper circle.

2. Sift the rice flour, cornflour, potato flour, cocoa, baking powder, baking soda and xanthan gum three times into a large bowl (or whisk in the bowl until well combined).

3. Whisk the eggs and caster sugar together in a medium bowl until thick and foamy. Add the melted butter, yogurt and milk and stir until well combined. Add to the dry ingredients and beat with a wooden spoon for 2 to 3 minutes, until well combined with no lumps.

4. Pour the batter into the tin and bake for 45 to 55 minutes, until firm to the touch (a toothpick inserted in the centre should come out clean).

5. Cool in the tin for 10 minutes, then remove the outer ring and turn out onto a wire rack to cool completely.

6. To make the chocolate icing, sift the icing sugar and cocoa into a bowl. Add the butter and milk and mix until well combined. Spread evenly over the cooled cake

PER SERVING (¹⁄₁₂ recipe, including icing): 386 calories; 5 g protein; 12 g total fat; 7 g saturated fat; 69 g carbohydrates; 2 g fibre; 206 mg sodium

Non-stick cooking spray

170 g superfine white rice flour

75 g cornflour

90 g potato flour

70 g unsweetened cocoa powder

2 teaspoons gluten-free baking powder

1 teaspoon baking soda

1 teaspoon xanthan gum or guar gum

2 large eggs

330 g caster sugar

45 g unsalted butter, melted

200 g gluten-free low-fat vanilla yogurt

170 ml semi-skimmed milk, lactose-free milk or suitable plant-based milk

CHOCOLATE ICING

240 g icing sugar

2 to 3 heaped tablespoons unsweetened cocoa powder

105 g unsalted butter, at room temperature

60 ml semi-skimmed milk, lactose-free milk or suitable plant-based milk

Hazelnut–Sour Cream Cake with Blueberry Jam

SERVES 10–12

If you have gluten-free baking experience, you may be used to baking cakes with almond flour, but have you tried hazelnut flour? It has a warm, distinctive flavour and is the basis for this hard-to-resist cake. If you find hazelnut flour to be cost prohibitive or difficult to locate, almond flour is a suitable substitute.

1. Preheat the oven to 180°C. Grease two 22-cm cake tins with cooking spray and line with parchment paper circles.

2. Place the butter, caster sugar and vanilla in a large bowl and beat with a handheld electric mixer until thick, pale and creamy. Add the eggs one at a time, beating well between additions.

3. Sift the rice flour, soy flour, cornflour, cinnamon, baking soda, baking powder and xanthan gum three times into a medium bowl (or whisk in the bowl until well combined). Stir in the hazelnut flour.

4. Using a large metal spoon, gently fold the dry ingredients into the butter mixture in two parts, alternating with the sour cream. Spoon the batter evenly into the tins.

5. Bake for 35 to 40 minutes, until a toothpick inserted into the centre comes out clean. Cool in the tins for 10 minutes, then turn out onto a wire rack to cool completely.

6. To make the cream cheese filling, combine all the ingredients in a medium bowl and mix well.

7. Spread the jam over one of the cake layers, followed by just

Non-stick cooking spray

195 g unsalted butter, cut into cubes, at room temperature

330 g caster sugar

2 teaspoons vanilla extract

3 large eggs

100 g superfine white rice flour

30 g soy flour

35 g cornflour

1 teaspoon ground cinnamon

1 teaspoon baking soda

2 teaspoons gluten-free baking powder

1 teaspoon xanthan gum or guar gum

100 g hazelnut flour

250 g light sour cream

CREAM CHEESE FILLING

115 g reduced-fat cream cheese, at room temperature

50 g hazelnut flour

1 teaspoon ground cinnamon

110 g icing sugar

1 tablespoon plus 1 teaspoon fresh lemon juice

160 g blueberry jam, plus more for garnish

(recipe continues)

over half of the cream cheese filling. Top with the second cake layer and spread with the remaining cream cheese mixture. Garnish with dollops of blueberry jam.

PER SERVING ($\frac{1}{12}$ **recipe**): 475 calories; 8 g protein; 26 g total fat; 11 g saturated fat; 54 g carbohydrates; 2 g fibre; 253 mg sodium

---

NOTE: If you have lactose intolerance, this recipe is not suitable for you unless consumed in very small amounts. If you would like to enjoy a regular serving size, I recommend that you first take an adequate number of lactase enzyme tablets (available at pharmacies).

ACKNOWLEDGEMENTS

A HUGE THANK YOU to my super special family and friends, who have always encouraged me in my work on FODMAPs. I am immensely proud that the diet I developed has now spread around the world and is helping so many. I couldn't have stayed so focussed without your support, and I am eternally grateful. Special thanks to Mum, Dad, Linda, Gra, Ang, Don, Mark, Zoe, Joel, Emily, Nana B, Nana S, extended family, Caitlyn, Jodie, Rosie, Paul, Susannah, Rohan, Dylan, the Shepherd Works team, Celiac Victoria, and other dear work colleagues – I treasure you all. And to my beautiful fiancé Adam, thank you for welcoming me and my crazy, busy life so warmly into yours.

Sincere thanks to the amazing team at Penguin, who originally published this wonderful book, including Julie Gibbs (publisher), Cath Muscat (photography), Michelle Noerianto (styling), Peta Dent (home economist), Megan Pigott (shoot producer), Rachel Carter (editor) and Lantern Studio (design) – you have made these fabulous recipes bigger and better than ever. I just love this book! Thanks so very much.

To the US team – thank you for believing in FODMAPs and enthusiastically embracing a second low-FODMAP book with me. Enormous thanks to Molly Cavanaugh, without whom this could not have been a reality. Your interest and experience in this space has been much appreciated, thank you. Also thanks goes to the other wonderful folk at The Experiment: Matthew Lore (publisher), Sarah Schneider and Anne Rumberger (publicity and marketing) and Karen Giangreco (digital publishing manager). It has been a fantastic journey working with you all.

To my readers: you are, after all, what this is all about. I understand and respect how it is to live with a restricted diet. I hope that you see these recipes as a celebration of flavour and enjoy sharing them with your friends and family, without worrying about feeling unwell afterward. Bon appétit!

YOUR FOOD DIARY

WEEK _____

DAY	BREAKFAST	MIDMORNING SNACK	LUNCH

AFTERNOON SNACK	DINNER	EVENING SNACK	SYMPTOMS

YOUR FOOD DIARY

WEEK _____

DAY	BREAKFAST	MIDMORNING SNACK	LUNCH

AFTERNOON SNACK	DINNER	EVENING SNACK	SYMPTOMS

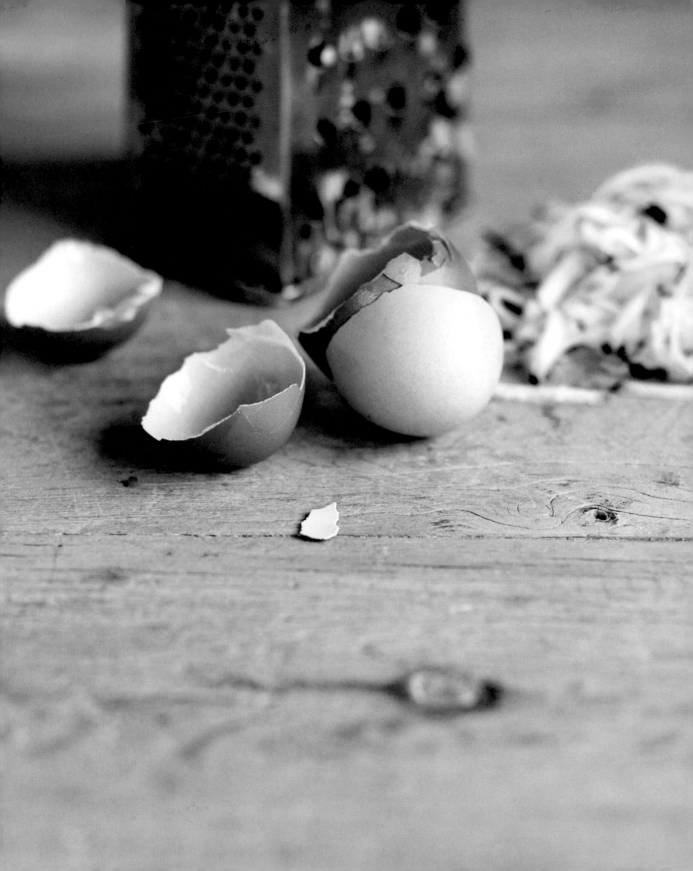

INDEX

Page numbers in *italics* refer to photos.

ABOUT THE AUTHOR

SUE SHEPHERD, PHD, is a dietitian who specialises in the treatment of dietary intolerances. She has a Bachelor of Applied Science in Health Promotion, a Masters in Nutrition and Dietetics and a PhD for her research into the low-FODMAP diet, coeliac disease and irritable bowel syndrome. Sue, who has coeliac disease herself, lives and breathes gluten-free and low-FODMAP.

For creating the low-FODMAP diet, a world-first scientifically proven diet for people with IBS, she was awarded the Telstra Australian Businesswoman of the year award, State Finalist (Victoria) award, 2013 *Financial Review*'s 100 Women of Influence in Australia Award, and the Gastroenterological Society of Australia's Young Investigator Award. She is the author of numerous peer-reviewed international medical journal publications, and is an invited speaker at international medical conferences as she is recognised internationally as an expert dietitian in the field of IBS and coeliac disease. She has authored thirteen cookbooks for people with coeliac disease, FODMAP intolerance and IBS, and runs Australia's largest dietitian private practice specialising in gastrointestinal nutrition, Shepherd Works.

She is the consultant dietitian on medical international advisory committees for gastrointestinal conditions, is on the editorial committee for Australia's leading health magazine, *Healthy Food Guide*, regularly consults to the media and was the resident dietitian on a national television programme. Sue is now a Senior Lecturer and Senior Researcher at the Department of Dietetics and Human Nutrition at La Trobe University in Melbourne, Australia, where she heads this department's research into FODMAPs. She also has a line of low-FODMAP food products.

SUE IS PROUD to head up Shepherd Works, Australia's longest-running gastrointestinal nutrition dietitian practice. Shepherd Works offers consultations to people who need education regarding the low-FODMAP diet and gluten-free diet, and dietary management for conditions such as IBS, coeliac disease, lactose intolerance, fructose malabsorption, Crohn's disease, ulcerative colitis and other digestive health issues. Sue and her team are committed to improving the quality of life for people with food intolerances and allergies, as well as increasing community awareness of these conditions. For more information, please visit www.shepherdworks.com.au.

Shepherd Works has several offices in Australia and offers Skype or telephone consultations for those who do not live nearby.